Medical Services and Consumer Protection in India

About the book...

This book is related to the investigation of patients' perception of medical services in India. It examines the implications of the application of Consumer Protection Act, 1986 to the medical services and its fall out on patient-doctor relationship. It also describes the existing legal measures pertaining to the redressal of patients' grievances against deficiency in medical services.

Furthermore, it evaluates the approach of the redressal agencies under the Act in deciding cases relating to deficiency in medical services. It also gives a review of various studies conducted in India and abroad on the subject of patients' perception of medical services.

About the author...

Renu Sobti obtained her B.Com. (H) degree from Hansraj College and M.Com., M.Phil. and Ph.D. degrees from the prestigious Department of Commerce, Delhi School of Economics, University of Delhi. Dr. Sobti is a Senior Lecturer in the Department of Commerce, Swami Shraddhanand College, University of Delhi.

She has published a number of articles in reputed journals of commerce and management and has also presented papers in conferences at national level. She is also the course co-ordinator of the distant learning programme for doctors on *Consumer Protection Act and Medical Negligence*, co-sponsored by Indian Medical Association and AKN Sinha Institute of Continuing Medical and Health Education and Research.

MEDICAL SERVICES AND CONSUMER PROTECTION IN INDIA

(Cases reviewed up to April 2001)

RENU SOBTI

NEW CENTURY PUBLICATIONS
DELHI INDIA
2001

New Century Publications
34, Gujranwala Town, Part-2,
Delhi - 110 033 INDIA
Tel.: 7247805, 7138192
Fax: +91-11-7464774
E-mail: indiatax@del2.vsnl.net.in

ICSSR Consultant: Dr. R.K. Mishra

First Published 2001

ISBN: 81-7708-011-3

This publication was partially financially supported by the ICSSR. The responsibility for the facts stated, opinions expressed, or conclusions reached, is entirely that of the author and that ICSSR accepts no responsibility for them.

Published by New Century Publications and printed at Print Line, New Delhi-110 002

PRINTED IN INDIA

Preface

The enactment of the Consumer Protection Act, 1986 was a milestone in the history of socio-economic legislations in India. The Act was passed to create awareness among the people regarding their legal rights as consumers and to protect them against unfair trade practices. The Act was amended in 1991 and 1993 to extend its coverage and scope and to enhance the powers of the redressal machinery.

The Act which applies to all goods and services (unless specifically exempted by the Central Government) and covers all the sectors whether private, public or co-operative, enshrines, *inter alia,* the following rights of consumers: (a) right to be protected against the marketing of goods and services which are hazardous to life and property, (b) right to be informed about the quality, quantity, potency, standard and price of goods or services, (c) right to be assured access to a variety of goods and services at competitive prices, (d) right to be heard and to be assured that consumer interest will receive due consideration at appropriate forums, (e) right to seek redressal against unfair trade practice or unscrupulous exploitation of consumers, and (f) right to consumer education. The Act also envisages establishment of consumer protection forums at the Central, State and District levels to provide a simple, speedy and inexpensive redressal of consumer grievances.

The historic judgement of the National Consumer Disputes Redressal Commission (National Commission) in 1992 that the medical services also constitute *service* under the Act, sparked off a country-wide controversy. Various High Courts and State Commissions held contradictory views on the issue. Finally, the controversy was laid to rest when the Supreme Court (in the *Indian Medical Association vs. V. P. Shantha case)* held in 1995 that medical services are covered under the Consumer Protection Act, 1986.

The judgement of the Supreme Court has wide implications for the patients as also for the doctors. Patients can expect improved quality of medical-care, compensation in case of negligence, inexpensive and speedy justice involving simple procedures. Conversely, possibilities exist for defensive medical practices, increased cost of treatment, refusal to attend serious cases and general deterioration in the 'humane' relationship between the doctor and the patient.

This study is related to the investigation of patients perception of medical services in India. It also examines the implications of the application of Consumer Protection Act, 1986 (CPA) to the medical services and its fall out on patient-doctor relationship. Furthermore, the study evaluates the approach of the redressal agencies under the Act in deciding cases relating to deficiency in medical services.

An attempt has been made to ascertain the views of doctors (in government and private hospitals and in private practice) and lawyers, judges, journalists and consumer activists on the issue.

The study is divided into six chapters.

Chapter 1 is introductory in nature and provides a conceptual framework and methodology of the study. It also reviews the major developments in patient-care across the world.

Chapter 2 gives a review of various studies conducted in India and abroad on the subject of patients' perception of medical services.

Chapter 3 describes the existing legal measures relating to the redressal of patients' grievances against deficiency in medical services, including relevant provisions of the CPA. Major cases decided by the National Consumer Disputes Redressal Commission and various State Consumer Disputes Redressal Commissions on medical negligence and deficiency in medical services have also been reviewed.

Chapters 4 and 5 are devoted to empirical investigations. The major findings of the survey conducted on patients to investigate into the patients' perception of medical services are discussed in

Chapter 4. Chapter 5 presents the major findings of the survey conducted on doctors and other experts on the subject to ascertain the implications of application of the CPA to medical services for the patient-doctor relationship.

Chapter 6 consolidates the major conclusions of the study.

I record my deep sense of gratitude to Professor D.P.S. Verma, Department of Commerce, Delhi School of Economics, University of Delhi, without whose help this study would not have taken its present shape. I am also grateful to Prof. Y.P. Singh, Head, Department of Commerce, Delhi School of Economics, University of Delhi and Dr. J.L. Bhat, Principal, Swami Shraddhanand College, University of Delhi for their encouragement and support.

I also express my thanks to Mr. H.D. Shourie, Director, Common Cause, Dr. N.K. Grover, Former President, Indian Medical Association and Dr. B.S. Negi, former Director of Research, Council for Social Development for their help and valuable comments.

I express my thanks to the Indian Council for Social Sciences Research (ICSSR), New Delhi for the publication grant and in particular Dr. A.P. Mangla, Head, Research and Publication Division, ICSSR and Dr. R.K. Mishra, Consultant ICSSR.

Dr. J.C. Sobti, my father-in-law, has been a constant source of inspiration and encouragement throughout the study. I take this opportunity to express my indebtedness to him. I owe a special word of appreciation to my husband, Mr. Kapil Sobti, and my daughters, Neharika and Riddhima, for many odds faced during the course of my study. Lastly, I must pay my gratitude to my parents, Late Shri A.S. Verma and Late Smt. Sheela Verma, as their blessings enabled me to complete my work.

Delhi
July 1, 2001

Renu Sobti

Contents

Preface

1. Medical Negligence and Consumer Protection: An Introduction **1-45**

1.1 Medical Services and Health
1.2 Consumer Protection in Medical Services
1.3 Conceptual Framework and Developments in Patient Care
1.3.1 Patient-Doctor Relationship
1.3.1.1 An Implied Contract
1.3.1.2 Fiduciary Concept
1.3.1.3 A Partnership
1.3.1.4 A Legal Contract
1.3.1.5 Ethical Aspect
1.3.1.6 Change in Relationship
1.3.2 Medical Negligence
1.3.2.1 Major Types of Medical Negligence
1.3.2.2 How to Prove Negligence?
1.3.3 Consent
1.3.4 Deficiency in Medical Services
1.3.5 Perception
1.3.6 Service Quality
1.3.7 Patient Satisfaction
1.4 Developments in Patient Care and International Trends in Consumer Protection
1.4.1 Developments in Patient Care
1.4.1.1 Patient-centred Approach
1.4.1.2 Medical Audit
1.4.1.3 Quality Control Circle
1.4.1.4 Medical Ombudsman
1.4.1.5 No fault Compensation Programme
1.4.1.6 Patients' Charter

1.4.2 International Trends in Consumer Protection
1.5 Conclusion

2. Studies on Medical Services: Global and Indian Experiences **46-58**
2.1 Studies Conducted Outside India
2.1.1 Studies Based on Patients' Perception
2.1.2 Studies on Quality of Patient Care
2.1.3 Studies on Patients' Satisfaction
2.1.4 Studies on Factors Influencing Physician's Choice
2.1.5 Study on Patients' Complaining Behaviour
2.1.6 Studies on Practice of Defensive Medicine
2.2 Studies Conducted in India
2.2.1 Studies Based on Patients' Satisfaction
2.2.2 Study on CPA's Benefits to Consumers
2.2.3 Studies on Consumers' Awareness of CPA
2.2.4 Study on Professional Indemnity Insurance
2.3 Conclusion

3. Medical Services in India: Regulatory Measures **59-210**
3.1 Relevant Provisions of the Indian Contract Act, 1872
3.2 Provisions of the Indian Penal Code, 1860
3.3 Relevant Provisions of the Law of Torts
3.4 Relevant Provisions of the Indian Medical Council Act, 1956
3.5 The Consumer Protection Act, 1986 and Medical Services
3.5.1 Relevant Terms
3.5.2 Enforcement Machinery under the Consumer Protection Act
3.5.3 Machinery for Redressal of Consumer Disputes
3.5.4 Limitation Period

3.5.5 Time Limit of Disposal
3.5.6 Reliefs for Deficiency in Service
3.5.7 Action against Frivolous or Vexatious Complaints
3.5.8 Penalties
3.5.9 The Supreme Court Judgement in *Indian Medical Association v. V.P. Shantha*
3.5.10 Functioning of the Consumer Courts
3.5.11 Approach of the Consumer Courts
3.6 Conclusion

4. Patients' Perception of Medical Services in India 211-242
4.1 Profile of the Sample: Patients
4.2 Patient's Perception Regarding Medical Services
4.2.1 Reasons for Patients' Choice of a Health Institution
4.2.2 Patients' Expectations from Medical Profession
4.2.3 Patients' Opinion about the Services Rendered at OPD
4.2.4 Patients' Satisfaction with the Quality of Medical Services
4.2.5 Perception as to Behaviour of Staff of Health Institution
4.2.6 Information about Illness and Treatment Provided by Doctors
4.2.7 Perception as to the Necessity of Information Regarding Treatment
4.2.8 Patients' Satisfaction over Doctor's Response to Queries
4.2.9 Patients' Awareness about Grievance Redressal under CPA
4.2.10 Patients' Overall Satisfaction with Medical Services
4.2.11 Action Taken by Dissatisfied Patients

4.2.11.1 Patients Dissatisfied and Suffering Specific Damages
4.2.11.2 Aggrieved Patients Needing Compensation
4.2.11.3 Action Taken by Patients Suffering Damages
4.2.11.4 Patients' Satisfaction with Remedial Measures
4.2.11.5 Action Proposed by Patients Dissatisfied with Remedial Measures
4.2.12 Perceived Injustice to Patients by Doctors
4.2.13 Perception Regarding Doctors' Professional Accountability
4.2.14 Patients' Grievances against Doctors and Health Institutions
4.2.15 Perception Regarding CPA's Role for Grievance Redressal
4.2.16 Indoor Patients' Perception: Additional Aspects
4.2.17 Perception of Patients Having Undergone Surgery: Additional Aspects
4.3 Conclusion

5. Grievance Redressal under Consumer Protection Act **243-268**
5.1 Profile of the Sample: Doctors
5.2 Profile of the Sample: Experts
5.3 Viewpoints of the Doctors' and Experts About Medical Services
5.3.1 Perceived Injustice to Patients by Doctors
5.3.2 Perception Regarding Doctors' Professional Accountability
5.3.3 Patients' Grievances against Doctors and Health Institutions

5.3.4 Awareness about Avenues for Action against Deficiency in Medical Services
5.3.5 Existing Legal Measures for Grievance Redressal
5.3.6 Perception Regarding Inclusion of Free Medical Services under CPA
5.3.7 Perception Regarding Redressal Mechanism under the CPA
5.3.8 Perception Regarding Basis of Patient-Doctor Relationship
5.3.9 Effect of CPA on Patient-Doctor Relationship
5.3.10 Effect of CPA on Quality of Medical Services
5.3.11 Implications of Application of CPA to Medical Services for Patient-doctor Relationship
5.3.12 Perception Regarding CPA's Role in Grievance Redressal of Patients
5.3.13 Doctors' Views on Additional Aspects
5.4 Conclusion

6. Conclusions **269-288**
6.1 Approach of Consumer Courts under CPA
6.2 Patient's Perception of Medical Services and Grievance Redressal under CPA
6.2.1 Patients' Satisfaction with Medical Services
6.2.2 Reasons for Patients' Dissatisfaction
6.2.3 Communication of Information about Line of Treatment
6.2.4 Accountability of Doctors
6.2.5 Factors Affecting Patients' Choice of a Hospital
6.2.6 Patients' Expectations from Medical

Profession
6.2.7 Perception about Performance of Duties by Doctors
6.2.8 Action Desired to be Taken by Dissatisfied Patients
6.2.9 Patients' Awareness of CPA
6.3 Doctors' and Experts' Viewpoints: CPA as a Means of Grievance Redressal Against Deficiency in Medical Services
6.3.1 Awareness of Regulatory Measures for Medical Services
6.3.2 Desirability of Inclusion of Free Medical Services under the CPA
6.3.3 Redressal Mechanism under the CPA
6.3.4 Quality of Medical Service Provided and the CPA
6.3.5 Perception about the Basis of Patient-Doctor Relationship
6.3.6 Necessity of Continuing Medical Education
6.3.7 Maintenance of Adequate Patient's Record
6.3.8 Implications of Application of CPA to Medical Services for Patient-Doctor Relationship
6.4 CPA's Relevance for Patient's Grievance Redressal

Appendices **289-302**
Bibliography **303-318**
Index **319-320**

Chapter 1

Medical Negligence and Consumer Protection: An Introduction

Health is considered to be man's most valuable possession since all his activities are influenced by the state of his health. Health has been defined by the World Health Organisation (WHO) as a state of complete physical, mental, and social well-being and not merely the absence of disease or infirmity. Disease implies absence of ease or comfort. According to Chambers Twentieth Century Dictionary [1], the meaning of the word disease is "uneasiness or a disorder or want of health in mind or body or ailment."

1.1 Medical Services and Health

The profession of medicine has immensely benefited mankind through restoration of good health. According to the New International Webster's Comprehensive Dictionary of the English Language [2], medical service means assistance or benefit pertaining to medicine or its practice offered to another, i.e., the performance of healing art or the science of preservation of health and of treating disease for the purpose of cure. It should be clear, therefore, that medical services imply delivering quality medical care to the community (i.e. service of mankind), in treating and curing afflictions of the human body.

The medical services include herein the services rendered by the hospitals (both government and private), nursing homes, health centres, clinics, medical practitioners (physicians, surgeons, and those practicing ayurvedic, homeopathic or any other system of medicine or surgery), chemists, diagnostic centers, paramedical staff, nursing staff, and other allied staff.

The question of professional duty to take care of health has assumed immense significance in the present day world. The

WHO is committed to provide health for all by the year 2000. The Directive Principles of State Policy under the Constitution of India require the State to make effective provision for public health, and for just and humane conditions of work [3]. It is the primary duty of the State to raise the level of nutrition, the standard of living of its people and the improvement of public health [4]. The Supreme Court has declared that right to medical aid is an integral part of right to life. It is an obligation on the State to preserve life by extending required medical assistance. In fact, the Apex Court has held that right to health and medical care is a fundamental right under the Constitution of India [5].

Practice of medicine is capable of rendering great service to the society provided due care, sincerity, efficiency and skill are observed by doctors. The word *doctor* is derived from the Latin word *docere* which means to teach. The doctor is a teacher who guides his patients about how to maintain positive health, prevent disease and treat it when the need arises. According to the New International Webster's Comprehensive Dictionary of the English Language, doctor means a qualified practitioner of medicine or surgery in any of its branches and patient means a person undergoing treatment for diseases or injury [6].

Doctors need scientific knowledge, technical skill and above all human understanding. Those who use these with courage, with humility, with wisdom and in accordance with medical ethics provide a unique service to their fellow men and women, and build an enduring edifice of character within themselves [7]. It is, therefore, a noble profession. Traditionally, the family doctor was considered to be a *friend, philosopher, and guide* for the sick. The relationship between the patient and the doctor was considered to be very sacred; it was based on mutual trust and faith, and it was not mercenary. According to Voluntary Health Association of India, the present state of medical profession seems to mirror the rot which seems to have set into our system [8]. Increased mechanisation and commercialisation of the profession has brought in an element of dehumanisation in medical practice [9].

Health care has now been reduced to a business which determines the patient-doctor relationship [10]. It is in this context that the question of consumer protection has become significant in the medical profession.

1.2 Consumer Protection in Medical Services

The consumer movement is gaining momentum across the world, in all spheres covering both goods or services. With increasing public awareness about their rights, the patients as consumers now insist on getting their money's worth in terms of quality health care [11]. The theme for the World Consumer Rights Day, celebrated on March 15, 1989, was "the Right to Responsible Health Care."[12].

Justice V. Balakrishna Eradi, President, National Consumer Disputes Redressal Commission, on April 21, 1992, delivered a landmark judgement [13] in the history of medical profession in India in which it was held that the patient is a *consumer* under Section 2(1)(d) of the Consumer Protection Act, 1986, and hence, entitled to invoke the jurisdiction of the redressal fora and that the activity of the opposite party (hospitals and doctors) constitute *service* as defined under Section 2(1)(o) of the Act, since *consideration* has been paid by the patient to the hospital for availing the services. It was also held that the legal heirs of the deceased are also considered as consumers and they are covered under this Act.

The judgement of the National Commission sparked off a country-wide controversy. While some people were in favour of the decision and asked for inclusion of even free medical services provided by government hospitals to be within the purview of the Consumer Protection Act, 1986, others criticized the decision. The issue was extensively debated upon in the media, in technical scientific journals (medical and non-medical), and in seminars and conferences. There was also a considerable debate on the impact of the implementation of the CPA to medical services on the patient-doctor relationship. The entire medical profession was disturbed by the judgement of the National Commission. The Indian Medical Association (IMA) vigorously opposed it [14]. Members of the medical profession were of the view that if the medical services come under the CPA, the patient-doctor relationship would be affected [15]; doctors would always be in a state of fear psychosis. They would then ask their patients to go in for all sorts of investigations, consultation, and would take medical indemnity insurance, which would mean considerable increase in cost of treatment and this would invariably be a burden on the patient [16]. Since under this Act patients are likely to proceed against doctors in courts of law. doctors would decline to accept high-risk cases for treatment, thus denying medical care to the really needy patients [17].

The arguments given in favour were that it was in this forum that a victim could get compensation [18]; and that the medical profession has became totally commercialised [19] and it was no longer a noble profession [20] and the medical professionals were conducting themselves without any sense of fear of liability against negligence and malpractice [21] and that the doctors were increasingly indulging in malpractice [22].

Even the various High Courts and the State Commissions were having different views on this aspect. In certain cases it was held that medical services are covered under the Act [23] whereas the contrary view was that such services are not covered under the Act [24].

Finally, the matter went to the Supreme Court, and its landmark judgement in the case of *Indian Medical Association vs. V.P Shantha*,[25] on November 13, 1995, brought the whole debate to a close. It affirmed that the services rendered to a patient, both medicinal and surgical, are covered under the Consumer Protection Act, 1986. It is thus, that the entire medical profession has come under the purview of the CPA.

The Supreme Court expressly made certain guidelines in the said landmark judgement to ascertain which services are covered and which are excluded. However, broadly speaking, the Medical

Services are covered under the provisions of Act if they are not free services.

The judgement of the Supreme Court is expected to have major repercussions. On the one hand, there are possibilities of benefits in the form of speedy decisions, in-expensive justice, simple procedures, relief to the victim in the form of compensation, improved quality of patient care and doctors becoming more careful. On the other hand, there are possibilities of adverse effects which include increased cost of treatment, defensive medical practice, refusal to attend serious patients, especially in case of emergency, and deterioration in the 'humane' relationship between the doctor and the patient.

The claims for damages in the cases of Medical Negligence, prior to the present enactment of the Consumer Protection Act, 1986, were maintainable in the civil courts under the provisions of the Law of Torts. The enactment of the present Act have provided a concurrent machinery to deal with the cases where there is an allegation of Medical Negligence or deficiency in service. The proceedings under the Act are speedy in nature in comparison to Civil cases and that too without any court fees. The enactment of the present Act has not taken away the jurisdiction of the Civil Courts but has provided an alternate remedy. Hence, the provisions of the Act provide a forum to the actual victims of medical negligence or deficiency in medical services by providing cheap, speedy and efficacious remedy to claim compensation.

1.3 Conceptual Framework and Developments in Patient Care

We now discuss the following relevant concepts which include patient-doctor relationship, medical negligence, deficiency in medical services, perception, service quality and patient satisfaction.

1.3.1 Patient-Doctor Relationship: The patient-doctor relationship is central to the patient satisfaction and to positive health outcomes. The most crucial healing element is not medicine or surgery, but a patient-doctor relationship which provides hope, confidence and a healthy environment [26]. Effective communication between the doctor and the patient is a central clinical function. The relationship between the patient and the doctor should be based, primarily on faith, confidence and holistic approach.

1.3.1.1 An Implied Contract: The patient-doctor relationship is defined, all over the world, by 'Code of Medical Ethics', issued by the Medical Councils of the respective countries or on the basis of guidelines and recommendations issued by international medical organisations like the Commonwealth Medical Association, World Medical Association and World Health Organisation. The relationship of fidelity and mutual confidence accrues, at the time when doctor undertakes or assents to provide medical services. Therefore, the nexus between the doctor and the patient is, normally, the result of implied contract between them; seldom any formal agreement is made between them.

1.3.1.2 Fiduciary Concept: Originating in the Roman Law, the fiduciary concept applies to relationship in which one person entrusts the management of his property to a second person, wherein the second person is expected to work for the benefit of the first person without making profit unfairly.

The fiduciary concept has been applied to the patient-doctor relationship as patient care resembles managing a valuable trust [27]. It refers to doctor's commitment to promote the patient's vital medical interests which include prolonging life, relieving symptoms and restoring normal functions of the body [28]. The patient's request for help and the doctor's offer to give it initiate the patient-doctor relationship. The doctor, thereby, becomes a fiduciary or trustee for patient.

1.3.1.3 A Partnership: According to the British Medical Association, the relationship between a doctor and a patient is based on the concept of 'partnership and collaborative effort' [29]. Decisions should be made through frank discussion, in which the doctor's clinical expertise and the patient's individual needs and preferences are shared, to select the best treatment option. The patient's consent to be examined and to receive treatment is the trigger which allows the interchange to take place. The basic premise is that the treatment is undertaken as a result of patient being actively invited in deciding what is to be done to them.

According to Kenneth, et agricultural. [30] for a good patient-doctor relationship the doctor should be a good communicator as well as technically competent. The goal should be 'involved partnership' by telling the patients about the various options available for treatment and involving them in the decision-making process.

1.3.1.4 A Legal Contract: The relationship between the doctor and the patient is also legally recognised as that of a contractual nature because its foundation lies in a consent and a contract emerging therefrom. The consent in a contract between a doctor and a patient may be expressed or implied. A consent by a patient may either be given by himself or any person on his behalf.

A contractual patient-doctor relationship is established when the patient makes a request for medical examination, diagnosis, opinion, advice or treatment and the doctor undertakes to provide these. There are situations when a request by the patient is not necessary, for example, treatment of an infant, where the parents make the request or that of a victim of accident. The sanctity of such a relationship safeguards the interest of the patient, the doctor assuming all responsibility for providing health care. The doctor is supposed to take reasonable care, i.e. care which a doctor of his standing would take in that circumstances.

The patient has every right to terminate the relationship with his doctor at any time and seek the help of another. A reciprocal right rests with the doctor who, at any time, takes the help of a colleague or specialists in the best interest of his patient. The patient, in doubt, despite detailed explanation by his doctor about the nature of his illness and treatment advocated, can ask for a second medical opinion.

The patient is obliged to follow reasonable instructions of the doctor and participate and co-operate in the treatment and its further evaluation. Failure to do so may not allow him to hold the doctor responsible for any resultant damage [31]. At the same time, the doctor, too must not make any tall promises which he cannot keep, nor should he guarantee any cure because he may become liable for breach of contract.

The doctor himself can terminate the relationship when he feels that his knowledge and skills are limited with respect to treating the patient's condition or when he feels that the patient could be better treated elsewhere [32]. Non-payment of fees does not form the grounds for termination of such relationship as the contract between the doctor and the patient exists, irrespective of the payment of fees. The remedy, in such a situation lies in a suit, for recovery of the fees rather than the termination of services [33].

Thus, if a doctor fails to fulfill his obligations, he is guilty of breach of trust under the Law of Contract, and the patient is entitled to claim damages for loss suffered by him due to breach of contract, under Section 75 of the Indian Contract Act, 1872. Breach of contractual fiduciary duty also results in negligence on the part of the doctor under the Law of Torts.

1.3.1.5 Ethical Aspect: The word ethics, according to the English Dictionary, denotes a system of moral principles, a code of conduct recognised in response to a particular group culture, e.g., medical and legal. Ethics is a normative discipline, designed to secure orderliness in the lives of people, and seeks to restrain the sources of degradation, viz., greed, cruelty and selfishness. The rights, duties, commitments, obligations, judgements and actions of the individual, as a member of the society, come within the purview of ethics.

Medical ethics deals with issues where ethics and medicine interact with each other. Medicine deals with facts and with deductions to be drawn therefrom. Ethics deals with the norms to be observed in human touch. The question of medical ethics arises, when a medical situation warrants application of ethical norms. A code of medical ethics is now accepted within the medical profession. Medical ethics includes the professional responsibilities and obligations of doctors.

Code of Medical Ethics: The code of conduct for doctors is almost as old as the medical practice itself. The Babylonian laws of Hummarabi (2200 B.C.) not only laid down the manner in which doctor had to perform, but also the penalty if he failed. The Hippocratic Oath dates back to 5-4 B.C. Frederick II of the Holy Roman Empire laid down the laws to regulate medical practice in 1240-41 [34]. There are also Helsinki and Tokyo declarations dealing with different aspects of medical ethics.

The charter of College of Physicians of London incorporated in 1518, specifically provided for the College to take action against its members for malpractice by a fine of sixty pounds or fourteen days imprisonment. The civil liability of physicians arose out of an early rule laid in 1534 by the English Jurist Sir Anthony Fitzherbert that "It is the duty of every artifeer to exercise his art right and truly as he ought." [35].

Besides legal regulations, various codes of ethics have also been adopted by medical professionals to regulate their conduct. The American Medical Association came out with code of ethics in 1847, which has already undergone five revisions. Code writing continues to the modern days, the most recent was the International Code of Ethics, issued by the World Medical Association in 1948, which has already undergone two revisions, the latest one being in 1982 [36].

In India, the Medical Council of India prescribes the code of conduct for doctors as encoded in the "Code of Medical Ethics", in which duties of the doctors has been described. The relevant parts of the code has been reproduced in Appendix I.

The Medical Council of India (MCI) prescribes the standards of professional conduct and etiquette and also lays down the duties of physicians to their patients and to the profession at large. Proper implementation of ethical standards in medical practice plays an important role in protecting human rights. The MCI was constituted to enforce uniform minimum standards of qualification in medicine.

The code of medical ethics includes a declaration, given to each medical practitioner at the time of registration, asking them to pledge to dedicate their lives to the service of humanity. The code covers certain general principles, duties of physicians and their responsibilities and in case of breach of duties, the disciplinary action to which they themselves can be subjected.

The code of medical ethics performs multiple functions. It regulates the behaviour of doctors in the interest of patients and also keeps competition among doctors under control.

The medical profession in India seems to be in the grip of a severe crisis in terms of medical ethics. Anyone with first hand experience of the system of medical care in India would realise that medical ethics as encoded in a detailed 'Code of Medical Ethics in India' are rarely adhered to [37]. Further, the relationship between the patient and the doctor appears to be inherently unequal, the doctor being more qualified, the patient cannot decide what is required to cure his or her malady and which doctor and what treatment is the best. It is in this context that there is a need for a code of medical ethics, and that it should be implemented effectively. Unfortunately, it appears that this document remains only on paper [38]. It is time that the code of ethics is taken seriously by professionals and patients.

1.3.1.6 Change in Relationship: Practice of medicine is as ancient as the existence of human race. Originally the priest functioned as preacher, teacher, judge as well as healer. He was the first physician. With the passage of time this job of a physician graduated into an independent profession. In the earlier era 'physician' was treated as 'next to God'. Gradually, his social stature reduced from 'next to God' to a 'friend, philosopher and guide' and then to a 'respectable professional' and today, to a 'service provider to health consumers'. This downslide in the social position and esteem of physician seems to be the result of deterioration of social values, materialistic approach to life, commercialisation of medical profession, higher expectations and awareness of their rights and privileges by patients, and increasing consumer activism.

Earlier, the relationship between the doctor and the patient was considered very sacred. However, from the fifth decade of the 20th century, there has been an increasing amount of dissatisfaction among patients as evidenced by increasing number of doctors and their patients ending up in the law courts. Patients have now become better educated and informed about the nature of disease and treatment and perhaps, with justification, began to expect better results and more transparency in the treatment [39].

The consumer movement in the health care sector in India is, therefore, at the crossroads. On the one hand, public awareness has been increasing, while on the other, the standard of health care delivery has been deteriorating. The situation is complex in our country due to different disciplines of medicine which have been traditionally and historically practiced. Regulation of different disciplines of medicines is very important. However, this aspect has remained neglected over the years. A plethora of medical colleges, mostly ill-equipped and started on capitation fee has complicated the situation further [40]. The consumer is caught in a trap. On the one hand, he has to deal with the powerful combine of an ill-equipped, uncontrolled medical profession, defunct regulatory bodies, an overburdened legal system and on the other, he has to face a grim health situation and the maladies arising out of it [41].

With the emergence of major private hospitals and private nursing homes, the doctor does not belong to the patient; he belongs to the institution. With materialism replacing moral and spiritual values, the system of cuts and commissions by and large governs the medical profession [42]. Today, that divine relationship has been and is being changed to that of mostly mature relationship. The doctor offers service, the patient is a consumer and so, if there is any shortfall in the services being offered, the doctor should be held responsible for his own shortcomings.

In government hospitals, it is difficult to get proper care and attention because demand is more than supply and often, the doctors make it known to the patient that he should seek an appointment at their private clinic, if he is interested in speedy recovery [43].

Thus, medicine which is used to having a personal equation between the doctor and patient has become a high-tech profession, often devoid of human touch. The idea that the doctors are for the people sounds like an alien doctrine. The shift from holistic health care to health care business is evidently clear.

1.3.2 Medical Negligence: When a patient comes to doctor for care and the doctor accepts the same, an implied contract comes into effect and a duty of care arises. Medical negligence is the breach of duty owed by a doctor to his patients to exercise reasonable care and skills, resulting in some bodily, mental and in turn, financial loss. Thus, medical negligence is one category of civil wrongs or tort. According to the Concise Oxford Dictionary of Current English [44], negligence means lack of proper care and attention, carelessness or an act of carelessness.

In the case of *Laxman B. Joshi v. T.B. Godbole and Anr.* [45], the Supreme Court observed :

"Failure to exercise reasonable skill as per the general standards and prevalent situations is termed as medical negligence. Therefore, failure of cure, occurrence of infection, complication, even a death can not be taken in isolation and termed as medical negligence. Law does not expect each medical practitioner to exercise highest skills".

Thus, medical negligence means failure to act in accordance with the standards of a reasonably competent medical man at the time. According to British Medical Association [46], negligence is the breach of a duty to use reasonable care as a result of which there is damage to another. In order to prove negligence, the aggrieved consumer must be able to establish to the satisfaction of the Court that :

1. The doctor owed him duty of care of a particular standard of professional conduct,
2. The doctor breached that duty,
3. The patient suffered actual damage, and
4. The doctor's conduct was direct and proximate cause of damage.

The standard of care in legal parlance has normally been assessed by the parameters of 'reasonable care and skill' and therefore, professional negligence, in case of doctors, has often been described as 'lack of reasonable care and skill' whereby the health or life of a patient is endangered [47].

Undertaking an assignment beyond one's competence is a gross case of rashness. Rashness arises because the doctor neglects his duty to be careful about the patient's safety and hence the term negligence can be used generally to cover both rashness and negligence.

In *M. Arunachala Vadivel and Ors. v. Dr. N. Gopala Krishnan* [48], medical negligence was defined as want of reasonable degree of care and skill or wilful negligence on the part of medical practitioners in the treatment of a patient with whom relationship of professional attendant is established so as to lead to his bodily injury or permanent disability or loss of life.

Thus, medical negligence is defined as lack of reasonable care and skill, or wilful neglect on the part of a doctor in the treatment of a patient, whereby the health or life of a patient is endangered.

Duty to Exercise Reasonable Skill and Care: Such a duty exists from the moment of establishing a patient-doctor relationship, that is, from the moment a patient approaches the doctor and the doctor examines the patient. Legally, this is also applicable in cases, where a doctor approaches an injured patient in a roadside accident and even if the patient is unconscious and totally unaware of the doctor's presence.

Therefore, the relationship need not necessarily be a contractual one but, may also arise when a doctor accepts or undertakes to treat a patient. The doctor, then owes a duty to the patient to use diligence, care, knowledge, skill and caution in administering the treatment.

Thus, the most important duty of the physician is to exercise reasonable skill, care and diligence throughout the treatment and in after-care. This duty to observe reasonable standard of care is not affected even if he renders the services gratuitously.

In *Laxman B. Joshi v. T. B. Godbole and Anr.*[49], the Supreme Court observed :

"The duties which a doctor owes to his patients are clear. A person who holds himself out, ready to give medical advice and treatment impliedly undertakes that he is possessed of skill and knowledge for the purpose. Such a person, who consulted by a patient owes him certain duties, viz., a duty of care in deciding whether to undertake the case, a duty of care in deciding what treatment to give, and a duty of care in the administration of that treatment. A breach of any of those duties gives a right of action for negligence to the patient. The practitioner must bring to his task a reasonable degree of skill and knowledge and must exercise a reasonable degree of care. Neither the very highest nor a very low degree of care and competence judged in the light of the particular circumstances of each case is what law requires".

The standard of care is flexible and adaptable to the circumstances because the same standard of skill and competence cannot be expected from every doctor; that is why the standard of reasonable care cannot be defined with mathematical precision. Standard of reasonable skill and competence is variable, depending upon the qualifications and experience of the doctor. Naturally, a higher standard of care is expected of a specialist due to his higher qualifications.

Thus, the yardstick is the degree of care which may be reasonably expected of a practitioner of average skill depending upon the actual circumstances of the case. In *Hucks v. Cole* [50], Justice Lord Denning made a very pertinent observation about standard of care :

"A doctor was not to be held negligent simply because something went wrong. He was not liable for mischance or misadventure or for an error of judgement. He was not liable for taking one choice out of two or for favouring one school rather than another. He was only liable when he fell below the standard of a reasonable competent practitioner in his field so much so that his conduct might be deserving of censure or inexcusable."

Thus, if the doctor does not bring the ordinary skills and knowledge, expected of a doctor of his standing to the care of the patient, then there is negligence. Further, an error of judgement by itself does not amount to negligence provided that the doctor possesses a reasonable degree of proficiency and has applied that proficiency with sufficient degree of diligence [*White House v. Jordon*] [51].

In *Vinitha Ashok v. Lakshmi Hospital and Others* [52]., the National Commission observed :

"The Law does not require that a doctor in the discharge of his duty of a case should use the highest degree of skill. Since that may never be acquired, it is enough for the doctor to show that he acted in accordance with the general and approved practice. A mistaken diagnosis is not necessarily a negligent diagnosis. A practitioner can be held liable in this respect only if his diagnosis is so palpably wrong as to prove negligence, that is to say if his mistake is of such a nature as to imply an absence of reasonable skill and care in the profession".

Thus, every person who enters the profession, undertakes to bring to the exercise of it a reasonable degree of care and skill. It is true that a doctor or a surgeon does not undertake that he will positively cure a patient nor does he undertake to use the highest possible degree of skill, as there may be persons more learned and skilled than him, but he definitely undertakes to use a fair, reasonable and competent degree of skill in the light of the circumstances of that case.

In *Bolam v. Friern Hospital Management Committee* [53], Justice McNair, while addressing the jury, summed up the law as under :

"The test is the standard of the ordinary skilled man exercising and professing to have that special skill. A man need not possess the highest expert skill; it is well established law that it is sufficient if he exercises the ordinary skill of an ordinary competent man exercising that particular art. In the case of a medical man, negligence means failure to act in accordance with the standards of reasonably competent medical men at the time. There may be one or more perfectly proper standards, and if he conforms with one of these proper standards, then he is not negligent."

"Negligence means failure to act in accordance with the standards of reasonably competent medical men at the time".

"A doctor is not guilty of negligence if he has acted in accordance with the practice accepted as proper by a responsible body of medical men skilled in that particular art .... Putting in the other way round, a doctor is not negligent, if he is acting in accordance with such a practice, merely because there is a body of opinion that takes a contrary view."

This decision has since been approved by the House of Lords in *White House v. Jordon* [54]; *Maynard v. West Midlands Regional Health Authority* [55]; and *Sidaway v. Bathlem Royal Hospital* [56].

The test pointed out by Justice McNair covers the liability of a doctor in respect of his diagnosis, his liability to warn the patients of the risk inherent in the treatment and his liability in respect of the treatment.

In *K. Gracykutty v. Dr. Annamma Oommen and Anr.* [57], the Kerala State Commission made an observation on the duties of a medical practitioner :

"The duty of a medical practitioner is based on the fact that he is handling a human being which is likely to cause physical damage unless proper care and skill are applied. A physician who diagnoses and treats a person for a disease or a surgeon who performs an operation on a patient to remove or rectify a defect is presumably making an undertaking that he possesses the required skill and knowledge for the purpose. He is duty bound in two respects, viz., he owes a primary duty of care in deciding whether he should undertake the case and after having undertaken the case, the next duty cast on him is the duty of care in the administration of the treatment wherein he should use diligence, care, knowledge and caution. His failure to perform either of the above two duties, if proved, will offer reasonable and valid ground to foist negligence on him. He need not be expected to possess the highest or a very high standard nor should he have a very low standard only. The law requires fair and reasonable standard of care and competence".

Breach of Duty of Care: In an action for medical negligence it must be proved that the doctor did not discharge his duty to take reasonable care. Breach of duty to take care means omitting something which a reasonable man would do or doing something, he would not do. Thus, failure to take care is to be interpreted as a failure to exercise reasonable skill and competence, expected of an ordinary doctor of ordinary prudence.

Damage Suffered by Patient: A patient cannot sue a doctor in the absence of any damage, even though the doctor may have been negligent and the loss suffered by the patient should be measurable and compensated in terms of money. Following losses can be suffered by the patients:

1. Loss of earning due to enforced absence from work or a change in occupation resulting in reduction in wages.
2. Additional expenses incurred by the patient for the treatment of complication caused as a result of negligence.
3. Reduction in life expectancy of the patient.
4. Loss of a limb or a sense organ resulting in a change in the quality of life of the patient, causing mental trauma or physical pain and suffering.

5. Damages in cases of female patients resulting in sterility, disfigurement or disability of any kind.

6. Death of a patient resulting in a loss to the relatives in terms of potential earning power of the deceased, specially if he or she was the bread earner of the family.

For assessing damages, the pain, suffering and financial expenses incurred as a result of the injury are taken into account. Depending upon the circumstances past, present and anticipated loss of earning capacity and medical expenses directly attributable to the injury are included.

Direct Causation: The most important element in a case of negligence or a malpractice suit is that the patient must prove that the failure to take any action or negligent action by the physician was the direct cause of harm suffered by him. In most of the cases of negligence, 'facts speak for itself', doctrine is applicable such as foreign bodies like sponges and forceps retained within the body, operating on a wrong patient and on a wrong organ.

1.3.2.1 Major Types of Medical Negligence: These are of the following types.

1. Negligence in Diagnosis: A proper diagnosis of the illness is the first duty of a doctor. Mistaken diagnosis is not necessarily negligent diagnosis, unless the symptoms are so apparent that any reasonably competent and skilful physician could say that this is the disease. Hence, for every mistaken diagnosis, doctor is not to be held liable. He is liable where he fails to do according to reasonable standard of care.

2. Administration of Drugs: Doctors and nurses can be held liable for negligent administration of drugs, leading to death or injury, e.g. wrong drugs, adverse drug reactions, side-effects and failure to warn patients about the after-effects.

3.Consent of the Patient: In any treatment and surgical procedure or invasive intervention on the body, written informed consent of the patient or if patient is unable to give such a consent, some relative's consent is necessary, otherwise the doctor can be held liable.

4. Negligence in the Operation Theatre: A number of litigations originate from the operation theatre. Negligence can be due to the following :

Wrong operation.

Negligent administration of anaesthesia.

Unhygienic condition of operation theatre.

Use of non-sterile instruments.

Use of non-sterile fluids.

Injuries caused during operation (e.g. burns).

Leaving foreign bodies and instruments inside the body.

Negligent acts by nurses and para-medical staff.

1.3.2.2 How to Prove Negligence? The task of proving medical negligence rests with the person alleging it, hence the doctor need not to prove his innocence. An exception to this general rule that the burden of proof rests upon the plaintiff, is in cases where the facts are so obvious that the onus is shifted to doctor to prove that he was not negligent, e.g., amputation of wrong limb or wrong digit at operation, burning of skin caused by strong antiseptic solution, leaving swabs or surgical instruments inside the patient after an operation. The three conditions considered essential to make doctrine of *res ispa loquitar* (fact speaks for itself) are (i) the nature of injury suggesting by common knowledge or expert evidence that without negligence it does not occur; (ii) the doctor must be in exclusive control of instrumentalities; and (iii) the patient/attendant must not contribute to his own injury. Thus, the burden of proving negligence is on the opposite party i.e. on the complainants, they have to stand on their own feet and not to take benefit of any lacuna in the evidence of the opposite party [58].

Liabilities for Medical Negligence: These are of the following types.

1. Individual Liability: Individual members of the profession are personally liable for the consequences of their acts. This liability is almost always based on the principles of faults. To be liable, the person must have done something wrong or must have failed to do something that should have been done. Thus, doctors, nurses, technicians and other para-medical staff are individually liable for the wrong acts.

2. Vicarious Liability: As a general rule, a man is responsible or liable only for his own acts. But, there are circumstances in which a person is liable for the wrongs committed by others, "Let the master answer". Vicarious means arising out of a *vicar* or a deputy or an agent. Vicarious liability indicates liability out of an agent's, a deputy's or a substitute's wrongful actions or omissions of their duties, and not out of the doctor's or health institution's own wrongs. In the course of their professional duties, doctors often have to take the services of nurses, technicians and para-medical staff. Thus, the doctor (if he owns the institution or nursing home) or the health institution that engages the doctors and others has vicarious liability. This liability is applicable only for civil liability. There is no principle of employer's liability in criminal law. This is particularly applicable to hospitals and other healthcare institutions where the institution becomes answerable for the wrong acts of the doctors, nurses, technicians, radiographers and other para-medical staff.

The vicarious liability to compensate the victim for monetary loss or injury to the body or mind is based on the principle that whosoever puts another person in his place to do an act or class of acts for him or in his absence (however short that absence may be), necessarily leaves that agent or employee, agent or proxy to act for the principal doctor or master. For legal purposes, the principal or the master is also answerable for the wrong of the person so entrusted either in the manner of doing that thing or in doing that thing in a manner in which it ought not to have been done, provided that is done in the course of the employment or engagement [59].

The position in the context of the responsibility of hospital authorities was clarified by Justice Denning, [60] in *Roe v.*

Minister of Health :

"that the hospital authorities are responsible for the whole of their staff, not only the nurses and doctors, but also for the anaesthetists and the surgeons (exception of consultants and anaesthetists employed by patient himself), whether they are permanent or temporary, resident or visiting, whole-time or part-time. The reason is, even if they are not servants, they are the agents of the hospital to give the treatment".

Further, the Supreme Court in *Achutrao Harbhau Khoolwa v. State of Maharashtra* [61] has accepted the principle of vicarious liability of State and held that running of hospitals is not an exclusive function of the government and is not in exercise of its sovereign power. The government cannot claim sovereign immunity from its liability for torturous acts of its employees. In fact, this principle becomes quite relevant in determining the accountability of the government to pay damages.

There is one exception to the principle of vicarious liability. If the employee instead of doing what he is employed to do, does something beyond his assignment or duty, or does something which he cannot be said to have been possibly asked or authorised to do, then the master has no vicarious liability [62].

1.3.3 Consent: Another major and important thing to do for a doctor is to obtain proper consent of the patient/attendant/relative. The word 'consent' implies voluntary agreement, compliance or permission. According to Section 13 of the Indian Contract Act, two or more persons are said to 'consent' when they agree upon something in the same sense to be legally valid and when it is given, it must be intelligent and informed. For the purpose of clinical examination diagnosis and treatment consent can be given by any person who is conscious, mentally sound and is of and above twelve years of age as provided under sections 88 and 90 of the Indian Penal Code, 1860. Consent is taken under section 13 of the Indian Contract Act, 1872. This Act, however, also provides under section 11 that only those persons who are of and above 18 years of age are competent to enter into a contract.

Since doctor-patient relationship amounts to entering into a contract consent should be obtained, specially written consent, from parents/guardian of a patient who is below 18 years so that validity of the contract is not challengeable. Consent given under fear, or misrepresentation of facts, or by a person who is ignorant of the implications of the consent, or who is under 12 years of age is invalid (Sec. 90 I.P.C.). Obtaining of a consent will thus be a cornerstone of protection against litigation. Depending upon the circumstances in each case consent may be implied, expressed or informed.

Implied Consent: This is by far the most common variety of consent in both general practice and hospital practice. The fact that a patient comes to a doctor for an ailment implies that he is agreeable to medical examination in the general sense. This, however, does not imply consent to procedures more complex than inspection, palpation, percussion, auscultation and routine investigations like sonography. For other examinations, notably rectal and vaginal and withdrawal of blood for diagnostic purpose, express consent (oral or written) should be obtained. For more complicated diagnostic procedures, e.g., lumbar puncture, radiology, endoscopy, C.T. scan etc. express written consent should be obtained.

Express Consent: Anything other than the implied consent is express consent. This may be either oral or written. Express oral consent is obtained for relatively minor examinations or therapeutic procedures, preferably in the presence of a third party. Express written consent is to be obtained for: (i) all major diagnostic procedures, (ii) general anaesthesia, (iii) for surgical operations, (iv) intimate examinations, (v) examination for determining age, potency and virginity, and in medico-legal cases.

Informed Consent: The concept of informed consent has come to the fore in recent years and many actions have been brought by patients who alleged that they did not understand the nature of the medical procedure to which they gave consent. All information must be explained in comprehensible non-medical terms preferably in local language about the diagnosis, nature of treatment, risks involved, prospects of success, prognosis, if the procedure is not performed, and alternative methods of treatment.

The doctrine of 'informed consent' requires that before any person is subjected to any medical or surgical procedure, he must be informed about the risks of that procedure and its alternatives and the patient or his guardian must then consent to undergo that procedure and he must be competent to give that consent.

The informed consent is an integral part of a contract between the patient and the treating doctor. Failure to obtain an informed consent of the patient (by not forewarning the patient of certain inherent risks of the contemplated medical procedure) is actionable.

It may not be possible for the surgeon to explain all the probable complications that one could meet during any surgical procedure but the law expects the doctor to explain to the patient at least the most common or most likely complications that are observed during such procedure [63].

The doctrine of informed consent in the context of civil liability has not yet been codified in India. In the field of criminal law, Section 90 of the Indian Penal Code (IPC) provides what is not consent. According to Section 90 [64], "A consent is not a consent as is intended by any Section and is given by a person under fear or injury, or under a misconception of facts, and if the person doing the acts knows or has a reason to believe that the consent was given in consequences of such fear of misconception."

The doctor's duty to disclose can encompass only those risks which are known to him at the time of administering the treatment [65].

Thus, it is the physician's duty to inform patient in comprehensive non-medical terms (preferably in local language) about the diagnosis, nature of treatment, risks involved, prospects of success, prognosis if the procedure is not performed and the alternative methods of treatment.

In *Dr. T.T. Thomas v. Elisa* [66], the Kerala High Court observed: "Consent is implicit in case of a patient who submits to the doctor and the absence of consent must be made out by the person alleging it. A surgeon who failed to perform emergency operation must prove with sufficient evidence that the patient refused to undergo the operation not only at the initial stage, but even after the patient was informed about the dangerous consequences of not undergoing the operation".

Relying on the aforesaid judgement in *K. Gracy Kutty v. Dr. Annamma and Anr.* [67] the Kerala State Commission held :

"It is a settled law that except in exceptional circumstances, a patient ought to be informed of the treatment that is proposed and his consent to seek treatment is obtained".

Proxy Consent: All the above types of consent can take the shape of proxy consent e.g. Parent for child, close relative for mentally unsound/unconscious patient, etc.

1.3.4 Deficiency in Medical Services: The Supreme Court, in a landmark judgment given on November 13, 1995, in the case of *Indian Medical Association v. V. P. Shantha* [68] held that patients who received deficient services by the medical profession and hospitals, were entitled to claim damages under the Consumer Protection Act, 1986.

Before the Consumer Protection Act, 1986, came into existence the term 'negligence' was used for dealing with failures or misdeeds of the doctors. In the Consumer Protection Act 1986, the term 'deficiency' has been introduced and defined under Section 2(1)(g).

Deficiency means any fault, imperfection, shortcoming and inadequacy in the quality, nature and manner of performance of any service. The Supreme Court further held that determination about deficiency in service was to be made, by applying the same test as was applied in an action for damages for medical negligence.

Medical professionals are expected to exercise or provide

reasonable degree of care in treating patients. A medical man rendering professional service for consideration is liable under the Consumer Forum, if he fails short of the standard of reasonably skilled medical person in the field. The Court did not accept the submission that deficiency in service rendered by medical practitioners could not be judged on the basis of any fixed norms and hence could not be covered under the Consumer Protection Act. Thus, the definition of deficiency under the CPA casts the net very wide and undoubtedly includes what is negligence in the law of tort.

The remedy for negligence differs from deficiency. A complainant can get compensation for loss or injury only in the case of negligence. Section 14(1) (d) of the Act indicates that compensation to be awarded is for the loss or injury suffered by the consumer due to negligence of opposite party. However, the other reliefs under the CPA can only be granted in the case of deficiency, such as removal of deficiency in services, refund of charges and provision of costs.

Negligence has not been defined in the Consumer Protection Act. The word 'negligence' has been indicated in Section 14(1)(d) of the Act. The Haryana High Court [69] has observed that the deficiency under CPA undoubtedly includes what is negligence in the law of torts, but it is somewhat wider. Thus, in all cases of negligence, there will be deficiency, but in all cases of deficiency, negligence will not be present. Deficiency may be the result of inability and lack of competence whereas negligence would be caused by carelessness and indifference.

1.3.5 Perception: Perception is the process by which an individual receives stimuli and gives them meaning, based on his previous learning memories, expectations, fantasies, beliefs, attitudes and personality. Thus, perception can be defined as "how we see the world around us".

According to Oxford Advance Learner's Dictionary of Current English, perception is "the process by which we become aware of changes through the senses of sight, hearing, smell, touch and taste." Kotler (1997) [70] defined perception as the process by which an individual selects, organises and interprets information inputs to create a meaningful picture of the world. Perception depends not on the physical stimuli, but also on the stimuli's relation to the surrounding field and on conditions within the individual.

Individuals act and react on the basis of their perception and not on the basis of objective reality. Thus, consumers' or patients' perception of health services is more important to a healthcare marketer than is their knowledge of objective reality. How people behave depends upon how they perceive the world around them.

1.3.6 Service Quality: Efforts in defining and measuring quality have come largely from the goods sector where it means zero defects, i.e. doing it right the first time. Knowledge about goods' quality, however, is insufficient to have an understanding about the service quality, as service has three well documented characteristics : intangibility, heterogeneity and inseparability.

Woodside, et al. [71] defined service quality as the consumer's comparison between service expectations and service performance. They concluded that no single definition of service quality fits all circumstances or situations.

According to Bopp [72], a medical encounter achieves quality in perception when it meets or exceeds the patients' expectations. Therefore, hospital marketers should concentrate on assessing patients' perception of quality.

From a service marketing perspective, a patient-centred approach is critical to the delivery of high quality medical services. For that purpose, quality must be defined by the patient not by the technical standard of service providers.

Kenneth, et al. [73] defined the quality from a service marketing perspective as the difference between patients' expectations prior to the service encounter and their perception of the service received. Clients will be dissatisfied with a service experience if it does not meet their expectations. Hence, patients' expectations serve as the foundation upon which medical service quality is evaluated by patients. It is the customer's definition of quality and not the management's definition that counts. Customers evaluate service quality by mentally comparing their perception of delivered services with their expectations of services [74]. When there is a discrepancy between customer's expectations, and management's understanding of customer expectations the perceived service quality suffers. Quality of care has become an essential issue to marketing of healthcare services. However, quality of care is difficult to define and even harder to measure.

Taylor and Cronin [75] (1994) viewed quality as a judgmental concept. According to them, "the real operational definition of quality is based on values and perception or attitudes".

Thus, quality can be described as meeting or exceeding customers' expectation. Today patients want value for their rupee; they don't want their rupees whisked away on things that are inappropriate, irrelevant, useless or potentially harmful.

Hospitals are also acknowledging that patients' satisfaction is of fundamental importance as a measure of quality of care. Thus, a multidimensional approach to measure healthcare quality focuses on access, image of healthcare personnel, clinical outcomes, patients' perception of health care and patients' satisfaction and out of these, patients' perception of healthcare and their satisfaction are the most important. Quality is a multi-dimensional construct and patients' satisfaction is the most important dimension [76].

1.3.7 Patient Satisfaction: Satisfaction is largely the result of fulfilled expectations of values. Turner and Louis [77] were of the view that satisfaction is a function of the perceived discrepancy of what an individual desires and what he or she actually experiences as a proportion of those desires. Desires were defined as expectations.

According to Woodside, et al.[78] patients' perception of service quality positively influences patient satisfaction, which, in turn positively influences the patient's decision to choose a specific health care provider. They defined patient satisfaction as a special form of consumer attitude, i.e. as a post-experience phenomenon reflecting how much a patient likes or dislikes the service.

According to Fisk, et al.[79], satisfaction results when service experience meets consumer expectations. Stimson and Webb [80] advocated that patient satisfaction was related to the perception of the outcome of care and the extent to which the outcome met expectation.

Taylor, S.A. (1994) [81] viewed service quality as a long term attitude that could be determined by measures of service from performance while patient satisfaction was a short term judgement of a service encounter and determined by measures that capture the gap between patients' perception of performance relative to their expectations.

Nelson, Carl W. (1990) [82] maintained that patient satisfaction could be determined by four variables, viz., satisfaction with outcome, continuity of care, patients' expectations and doctor-patient communication.

Thus, patient satisfaction is the result of fulfilled expectations of patients, which depends upon patients' perception of medical services received and the extent to which services received meets their expectations.

1.4 Developments in Patient Care and International Trends in Consumer Protection

This section is devoted to the developments which have taken place to improve patient care and the international trend on consumer protection against deficiency in medical services.

1.4.1 Developments in Patient Care: An account of major developments which have taken place to improve patient care are presented hereby

1.4.1.1 Patient-centred Approach: This approach encourages doctors to include patients as 'partners' in health care process. It encourages patients to ask questions, to seek a second opinion, and to share responsibility for medical decisions [83]. This approach requires effective doctor-patient communication.

The doctor-patient communication has been described as an integral component of quality medical care [84]. Poor communication on the part of the doctor is a major factor leading to patients' and relatives' dissatisfaction with care [85]. Frank communication with the patients and their relatives avoids many problems. A patient has the right to full information about diagnosis and treatment possibilities. In this approach, the doctor should give the necessary information in a way that is comprehensible to the patient, which is the cornerstone of developing better patient-doctor relationship. This approach requires that information should be formal, honest, decent and truthful [86].

In this approach, the patient must be well-informed in order to make health-care decisions and work intelligently in partnership with the doctor [87]. Effective patient-doctor communication can dispel uncertainty and fear and enhance healing and patient satisfaction.

In addition, this requires doctor to disclose to patients the information about procedural or judgement errors made in course of care, if such information significantly affects care of the patients[88].

1.4.1.2 Medical Audit: Medical audit is a method of objective evaluation of the quality of medical care. This is conducted by the service providers themselves (in house; the doctors and hospital administrators) supervised by a peer group. It facilitates self-assessment, by looking at current medical practices, comparing them with set standards of medical care and suggesting changes for implementation and improvements [89]. It helps detect deficiency in medical services provided, to improve attitude, skill and knowledge of the providers and to ensure collective responsibility and accountability.

Medical audit is designed to measure the care received by

patients as judged by established standards and criteria. The purpose is to identify both strengths and weaknesses of policies and procedures, and ultimately to correct deficiency or deviation from accepted standards [90].

Medical audit involves audit of structure, process, outcome, patient satisfaction, and cost. An effective medical audit system for improving health care facilities should have a performance parameter. The medical audit should help improve cost efficiency, consistency and quality of care as per the changing market demand in cases of quality ethics and the consumer laws.

The medical audit encourages doctors and nurses to coordinate their plans for patient care, improve their communication, identify needs for revision of policies and procedures and reassess equipment, personnel and other aspects of patient care.

1.4.1.3 Quality Control Circle: A quality control circle is a small group of usually eight to ten staff members who work in the same department under the same supervision. They meet voluntarily on a regular basis to identify, analyse and develop solution to problems in their specific work area. Each member must be committed to improve work methods, patient satisfaction, employee satisfaction and reduction in cost and be willing to work. This may require data collection and presentation to peers and management. Some problems can be solved directly by the circles, others can be presented to management with recommended solutions [91]. The circle evaluates the success of its solutions and it is committed to make them work. Documentation of quality control circle's activities becomes part of the overall hospital quality assurance program.

The operative precept in the concept of quality control circles (QCC) is "the man wearing the shoe knows best where it pinches", which means the employee working at the micro level is the one who is most familiar with the problems related to his work area. Therefore, the employees' innate familiarity and their ability are together used to find the solutions of the problems. In this process, congruence is made between the organisational and the individual goal.

Though many organisations in the manufacturing sector have adopted the concept of QCC, the State Bank of India, Bhopal Quality Circle has been the first instance of successful integration of the philosophy of QCC in a service industry [92]. The quality circles in banks have yielded results that are truly novel. The problems that the staff learnt to live with or had ignored hitherto, were solved. There has been an attitudinal metamorphosis among the members of QCCs. This radical transformation in the work ethics has manifested itself in more responsible behavioural patterns and improved services.

The health institutions can adopt this concept in order to improve the services provided to patients. Services provided by the health institutions cannot improve unless the employees at all level including the hospital administrators, doctors or other para-medical staff are deeply involved.

1.4.1.4 Medical Ombudsman: Creation of ombudsman would enable the consumers to have speedy and effective redressal of their complaints. This practice is being followed in the UK. The National Consumer Council (NCC) was set up in UK in 1975 [93] with a specified upper limit of compensation. If a consumer decides not to accept the decision he can still take legal action. The service provided by the ombudsman is free of charge and reviewed from time to time [94]. The system of ombudsman have been successfully adopted by a leading English daily in India [95].

The service of the ombudsman is useful to those consumers who are reluctant to take legal remedy because of the costs or delays of litigations or because of lack of familiarity with the law and the legal system or access to the legal services. Keeping in view that the Indian patients have the same reasons for not seeking redressal under the law, it is desirable that health institutions individually or collectively set up ombudsman to deal with disputes.

Having an ombudsman in India would not only give the hospitals the opportunity to redress the grievances of patients but also improve and maintain public confidence. It could provide health institutions with the valuable information about the causes of dissatisfaction amongst their patients, which enable them to improve their services. By this system, the burden of the legal system can be reduced and many of the complaints can be solved by the ombudsman.

1.4.1.5 *No fault* Compensation Programme: Under 'no fault' compensation programme[96], the objective is to provide a quick, cost-effective and fair means of compensating victims of medical accidents. The 'no-fault' prefix means that the victims do not have to prove in a court of law but to pursue the appropriate board that the damage has resulted from someone else's negligence and has occurred in circumstances which qualify within the conditions laid down by 'no-fault' scheme.

The 'no fault' prefix does not mean that it will no longer be necessary to investigate the reasons for a medical accident or to attribute blame for any blameworthy conduct which may have contributed to the damage caused by the accident. Indeed, it is an essential component of any 'no-fault' scheme for compensating victims of medical accidents that effective procedures should be followed to investigate the circumstances of such accidents including provisions for penalising doctors having acted carelessly in causing the accident. Under this the affected patients and his relation may be paid compensation without any inquest by the insurance companies from a fund equally contributed by patient, doctor, institution, and the government [97].

According to Harvard, one of the consequences of the introduction of a 'no fault' scheme is improvement in the chances of detecting careless and incompetent medical treatment [98].

As there are some whose injuries are highly significant but do not wish to pursue compensation because of the financial risks involved, would be willing to pursue the case under 'no fault' scheme.

The necessary condition for a claim to qualify under the 'no fault' scheme is whether the injury could have been prevented by an alternative diagnostic or medical procedure or by performing the procedure differently [99].

Havard [100] felt that the cost and the delays involved in the present law of torts created formidable obstacles and there was little prospects of any radical reform in it. Therefore, a properly constructed 'no-fault' compensation scheme offers a feasible alternative which would be acceptable to most of the victims.

In USA such a system has been introduced in the States of Virginia, Florida and New York. Sweden and Netherland in Europe and New Zealand have been practicing this 'no-fault' system for medical injuries since 1990 [101].

1.4.1.6 Patients' Charter: Citizens' charter is a comprehensive programme to raise quality, increase choice, secure better values and extend accountability. It can be modified to suit changing circumstances. The charter sees the services through the eyes of those who use them. It is a programme to raise the quality, extend accommodation, carry out the services fairly, effectively and courteously. The charter defines the minimum needs of the people which should be fulfilled [102].

The citizens' charter gives the citizen, published standards and results, choice and competition to improve quality, responsiveness and value for money to get the best possible service within the resources the nation can afford. This gives more power and freedom to the citizen to choose and also ensures that the citizens' voice is heard. The scheme of citizens' charter has been implemented in United Kingdom for all public services including National Health Services [103]. Citizens' charter in health services deals with requirements of the health services to be rendered to people or society.

In India, the National Consumer Council in 1994, made an expert group comprised of representative from consumer groups, the Indian Medical Association, and the Medical Council of India to develop 'patients' charter' which was notified by the Government of India in 1996 by the Ministry of Civil Supplies, Consumer Affairs and Public Distribution [104]. The 'patients' charter' specifies the rights and duties of the patient. The charter can be of immense help to patients if implemented properly.

1.4.2 International Trends in Consumer Protection: It is universally accepted in principle that the medical profession is morally, ethically and legally accountable to the patients in particular, and society in general. In most parts of the civilised world, the right of patients to receive compensation for injury is either accepted or appreciated. By and large, the Law of Torts is used to deal with the medical liability cases. In addition to the legal procedure (civil and criminal), the Medical Councils and the professional associations of the respective Countries, deal with the complaints against doctors and award judgement after proper inquest.

In Europe, the European Community Legislation has given a directive that the liability of suppliers of services be abandoned for the medical profession. Some progressive laws, like the Patients Injury Law, are also being considered to protect the interest of the patients without affecting the doctors [105].

In USA, 60 professional organisations making a coalition having representatives from medicine, law, pharmaceutical industry, media, church, and chambers of various trades have recommended radical amendments in the liability litigation laws to minimise defensive medical practice and its costs. They have also recommended that medical profession should have complete immunity from liability litigations. The fines should be paid in deferred instalments. They have further recommended that preferably a 'no fault-insurance' system should be introduced which has already been introduced in some states in USA, like New York, Virginia and also in many countries in Europe, including Sweden, Netherlands, Denmark and Norway [106].

In Australia, the Medical Council deals with all such cases through specific 'Tribunals' composed of peers abreast with latest treatment and with medical ethics and has duly laid that it will not accept any interference even by Kangaroo's Court [107]. The Australian Medical Council made it clear that only a tribunal such as medical board or similar bodies, capable of judging doctor's competence and in consonance with ethics, will hear such cases [108]. They are trying to evolve model doctor-patient relationship.

In Netherlands, while the government is preparing a 'Bill of patients' rights', the National Organisation of Consumers and the Royal Dutch Medical Association are collaborating in bringing about 'model' regulation to govern the patient-doctor relationship [109].

In Germany, the State Chambers of Physicians (a statutory organisation) have installed boards to deal with complaints of patients and to settle these without reference to Courts. Argentina, Austria, Belgium, Canada, Finland, Ireland, Israel, Malaysia, New Zealand, Sweden, UK and USA have no special laws other than the normal civil laws and procedures to deal with the malpractice liability claims [110].

In Hong Kong and Singapore, the consumer protection laws (the Consumer Council in Hong Kong and the Sale of Goods Act in Singapore) cover doctors and the services provided by the medical profession. In these two countries, the complaints against doctors are referred to the respective Medical Councils which are statutory bodies dealing with registrations, ethical practice and discipline of doctors, for settlement or arbitration, failing which the respective Medical Councils order inquest based on which the awards are given [111].

1.5 Conclusion

The patient-doctor relationship is based on mutual trust and faith. The British Medical Association advocated that it should be based on 'partnership and collaborative effort' and patients should be actively involved in the treatment process. The concept of medical negligence implies the breach of a duty of reasonable care as a result of which there is damage to the patient. Medical Negligence is a matter of major concern throughout the world. In order to avoid disputes, the doctor should always follow the doctrine of `informed consent'.

The term 'deficiency' has been defined under Section 2(1)(g) of the Consumer Protection Act, 1986. Earlier, the term negligence was used to cover the defaults of the doctors. `Deficiency' is a broader term and includes `negligence'.

The term perception implies "how we see the world around us". Service quality is the patients' expectations prior to service rendered and their perception after the service has been received. Health care institutions have started acknowledging that patient's satisfaction is of fundamental importance with regard to quality of care. Satisfaction is the result of fulfilled expectations of values. Thus, quality is a multidimensional construct and patient satisfaction is the most important dimension.

There have been considerable developments in patient care across the world and various countries are increasingly adopting the `patient-centred' approach and the `partnership' concept with a view to making the patient-doctor communication an integral component of quality medical care. The `patient-centred' approach, quality control circles, medical ombudsman, `no fault' compensation programme, and patients' charter should be adopted and implemented effectively by the health care organisations operating in India to improve the services provided to patients so that patients are satisfied with the services and chances of disputes are minimised.

Notes

1. Chambers Twentieth Century Dictionary, 1976 (New Delhi: Allied Publishers Ltd.), p.369.

2. The New International Webster's Comprehensive Dictionary of the English Language, 1995 (Chicago : J.G. Ferguson Publishing Co.),

p.791, 1149.

3. Articles 41 and 42 of the Constitution of India.

4. Article 47 of the Constitution of India.

5. See : Parmanand Katara v. Union of India, AIR 1989 SC 2039; Consumer Education and Research Centre v. Union of India, AIR 1995 SC 1922; State of Punjab v. Mahinder Singh Chawla, AIR 1997 SC 1225.

6. The New International Webster's Comprehensive Dictionary of the English Language, op cit, p.374.

7. The relevant parts of 'Code of Medical Ethics', as propounded by the Medical Council of India, have been given in Appendix I.

8. Voluntary Health Association of India (1992), Health for the Millions, Speciality issue on Consumer Action, Vol. 18, No.6 (December), p.1 (editorial).

9. Phatnani, Pitam, P. (1995), "Medico-Legal Aspects of Doctor-Patient Relationship", Express Pharma Pulse, November 30, p.5.

10. Mathew, N.M. (1995), "Consumer Talk", Health for the Millions, January–February, p.62.

11. Vaz, Walter (1996), "Copra-Primordial Prevention and Pre-emption", Indian Journal of Clinical Practice, speciality issue on Medilaw, May, p.35.

12. "Responsible Health Care : Every One's Right", Consumer Confrontation, Vol.9, No.1, (1989), pp.11–14 , 20 (Since renamed, Insight).

13. Cosmopolitan Hospital and Anr. v. Vasantha P. Nair (First Appeal No. 48 of 1991) and Cosmopolitan Hospital and Anr. v. V. P. Shantha and Ors. (First Appeal No. 94 of 1991) Consumer Protection

Judgements (CPJ), I (1992), CPJ 302 (NC).

14. IMA's Policy Document (1994), Consumer Protection Act vis-à-vis Medical Profession : Stand of Indian Medical Association, Indian Medical Association, New Delhi.

15. Ravindran, T.N.B. (1993), "Consumer Protection Act and Doctor", Souvenir, 69th All India Conference of Indian Medical Association, December, 25-30.

16. Chari, R.C. (1993), "More Menace than a Help to Health Professional", Health Action, Vol.6, No.6, pp.22-23; Grover, N.K. (1993), "Consumer Protection Act and Medical Profession", Delhi Medical Association News Bulletin, June 25, pp.7-12.

17. Goyal, R.C. (1992), "Is Patient a Consumer?", Health for the Millions, A Journal of Voluntary Health Association of India, Vol. 18, No.6, pp.25-28.

18. Saraf, D.N. (1992), "Genesis of Consumer Protection Act", Health for the Millions, Vol. 18, No.6, pp.21-24.

19. Jindal, R.P. (1993), "Doctors Heal Thyself", The Hindustan Times, March 3, p.13.

20. Mehta, P. (1992), "Do Doctors have a License to Kill?", Health for the Millions, Vol. 18, No.6, pp.7-10.

21. Saraf, D.N., op cit.

22. Bal, A. (1992), "Medical Councils : Failure to Enforce Code of Ethics", Health for the Millions, Vol.18, No.6, pp.11-14.

23. See : M/s Cosmopolitan Hospital & Anr. v. Smt. Vasantha P. Nair, I (1992) CPJ 302 (NC), Consumer Education and Research Society v. Dr. Rati Lal Patel & Ors., III (1992) CPJ 25 (NC); B. Shekhar Hedge v. Dr. Sudhanshu Bhattacharya & Anr., II (1992) CPJ 449; and Dr. G.C. Batalia v. The Consumer Disputes Redressal Forum & Anr., II (1994)

CPJ 523.

24. Dr. C.S. Subramanaram v. Kumarasamy and Anr., 1994 (3) CPR 403.

25. Indian Medical Association v. V.P. Shantha, III (1995) CPJ 1 SC.

26. Kenneth, E. Clow, et al. (1995), "Patients Expectations of Dental Services", Journal of Health Care Marketing (A Quarterly Publication of American Marketing Association), Vol.15, No.3 (Fall).

27. Ahmed, S.A. (1994), "The Fiduciary Concept : A Basis for an Ethics of Patient Care", Souvenir, Medimeet, 1994 (The 23rd Assam State Medical Conference of Indian Medical Association, 10-20 February, 1994, Nalbari, Assam).

28. Ibid.

29. British Medical Association (1993), Medical Ethics Today (London : BMJ Publishing Group), p.1.

30. Kenneth, E. Clow, op cit.

31. See : Md. Aslam v. Ideal Nursing Home, III (1997) CPJ 81 (NC).

32. Pandya, Sunil K. (1995), "Doctor-Patient Relationship", Medical Ethics, Vol.3, No.2 (April-June), p.23.

33. Phatnani, Pritam P. (1995), "Medico-legal Aspects of Doctor-Patient Relationship", Express Pharma Pulse, November, 30, p.6.

34. Kala, S. (1993), "The Doctors' Dilemma", Delhi Medical Association News Bulletin, July 10.

35. Sander, A.A. (1957), "The History of Professional Liability Suits in the United States" Journal of American Medical Association, Vol.163, No.6, pp.459-466.

36. Kala, S. (1993), op cit.

37. Jesani, Amar and Vimla Nandkani (1993) "Patients' Rights : A Perspective", The Indian Journal of Social Work (Tata Institute of Social Sciences), April, p.169.

38. Kohli, P.K. (1994), "CPA : Let Us Face It" Haryana Medical Journal, March-April, p.24.

39. Dayal, Arvind (1994), "Legal Aspects of Health Care", Indian Journal of Clinical Practice, Vol.8, No. 4 (January), p.68.

40. Bal, Arun (1993), "Consumer Protection Act and Medical Profession" , The Indian Journal of Social Work (Tata Institute of Social Sciences), April, pp. 209-210.

41. Ibid.

42. Mohan, Sadhana (1991), "Strong Medicine", The Times of India, February 16.

43. For details, see : Malhotra, Preeti (1996), "Hospitals : Gasping for Breath", The Hindustan Times (The Metropolitan), October 9, p.1; The Hindustan times (1997), "Doctors Leave Patients in Lurch", July 2; The Hindustan Times (1997), "Patients go through a Living Hell", January 21; The Hindustan Times (1997), "Here Patients are Left to their Fate", January 19; The Hindustan Times (1997), "Inhospitality Reigns Supreme Here" January 22; The Hindustan Times (1997), "Doctors Here 'Hand Over' Patients to God !", January 20; The Hindustan Times (1995) "Trans-Yamuna Healthcare Pathetic", February 27.

44. The Concise Oxford Dictionary of Current English (1990), 8th ed. (Oxford University Press), p.794.

45. AIR 1969 SC 128.

46. British Medical Association (1992), Rights and Responsibilities of Doctors (London : BMJ Publishing Group), p.19.

47. Parikh, C.K. (1990), Parikh's Text Book of Medical

Jurisprudence and Toxicology, 5th ed. (Bombay : CBS Publishers & Distributors), p. 574.

48. II (1992) CPJ 764.

49. AIR 1969 SC 128.

50. (1968) 118 New LJ 469.

51. (1980) I All ER 650.

52. II (1992) CPJ 372 (NC).

53. (1957) 2 All ER 118.

54. (1981) 1 All ER 267.

55. (1985) 1 All ER 635.

56. (1985) 1 All ER 643.

57. (1992) 1 CPR 251.

58. Harbhajan Singh Vs. Dayanand Medical College and Hospital & Ors. III (1996) CPJ 263.

59. Lele, R.D. (1992), The Medical Profession and the Law (Bombay : Sajjan Sons Publishers), p.16.

60. (1954) 2 All ER 136.

61. (1996) 4 CTJ 950 (SC).

62. Lele, R.D. (1992), op cit., p.17.

63. Save, Sudhakar and R.V. Govani (1999), "Informed Consent", Gujarat Medical Journal, Vol.56, No.1 (February), p.48.

64. Indian Penal Code, 1861, Section 90.

65. Save, Sudhakar et al., op cit, p.51.

66. AIR 1987 Ker. 52.

67. 1992 (1) CPR 251.

68. III (1995) CPJ 1 SC.

69. Dr. Ravinder Gupta v. Ganga Devi, 1993 (3) CPR 255.

70. Kotler, Philip (1997), Marketing Management :Analysis, Planning, Implementation and Control, 9th ed. (Delhi : Prentice Hall of India Pvt. Ltd.).

71. Woodside, A.G., L.L. Frey and R.T. Daly (1989), "Linking Service Quality, Customer Satisfaction and Behavioural Intention," Journal of Health Care Marketing, Vol.9, No.4, pp.5-17.

72. Bopp, K.D. (1990), "How Patients Evaluate the Quality of Ambulatory Medical Encounters : A Marketing Perspective," Journal of Health Care Marketing, Vol.10, No.1, pp.6-16.

73. Kenneth, E. Clow, et al. (1995), "Patient Expectation of Dental Services", Journal of Health Care Marketing, Vol.15, No.3.

74. Berry, L.L, A. Parasuraman and V.A. Zeithaml (1988), "Service-Quality Puzzle" Business Horizon, September-October.

75. Taylor, Steven. A. and Joseph J. Cronin (1994), "Modeling Patient Satisfaction and Service Quality" Journal of Health Care Marketing, Vol.14 (Spring), pp. 34-44.

76. Turner, Paul D. and G. Louis (1995) "Beyond Patient Satisfaction", Journal of Health Care Marketing (AMA), Vol.15, No.3 (Fall), pp. 45-51.

77. Ibid.

78. Woodside, et al., op cit.

79. Fisk, T.A., C.J. Brown, K. Cannizzairo, and B. Naftal (1990), "Creating Patients Satisfaction and Loyalty", Journal of Health Care Marketing, Vol.10, No.2, pp.5-15.

80. Stimson, G. and B. Web (1975), On Going to See the Doctor (London: Routledge and Kegan Paul).

81. Taylor, S.A. (1994) "Distinguishing Service Quality from Patient Satisfaction in Developing Healthcare Marketing Strategies". Hospital and Health Services Administration, Vol.39, No.2 (Summer), pp. 221-236.

82. Nelson, Carl, W. (1990) "Patient Satisfaction Survey : An Opportunity for Total Quality Improvement", Hospital and Health services Administration, Vol.35, No.3 (Fall), pp. 409-427.

83. Consumer Reports (1995),"How is Your Doctor Treating You ?", February, Vol.60, No.2, p.82.

84. World Health Organisation (1993), Doctor-Patient : Interaction and Communication : A Document (Switzerland :Division of Mental Health, WHO), p.1.

85. Ibid., p.2.

86. Navrange, Jayant (1994), "CPA and Doctors", Imates, Indian Medical Association, Pune branch, January,p.8.

87. American College of Physicians (1993), Ethics Manual, 3rd ed. (U.S.A.: American College of Physicians), p.9.

88. Ibid.

89. Mathew, N.M.(1987), "Quality Health Care : A Mirage or Reality?", Health for the Millions, March-April, P.39.

90. Purkayastha, P.K. (1993), "Liability and Accountability : With Reference to Operating Room Technique", Health Administrator, Vol.4, No.2 (December), p.128.

91. Ibid.

92. Sinha, M.K. (1986), "Quality Circle in Banks : The Bhopal Circle Experience", State Bank of India Monthly Review, December, p.584.

93. Metha, R.R.S. (1988), "Personal Banking Services : UK Examples", Prajnan, June, pp. 235-239.

94. Lamont, Linda, (1994), "When Things Go Wrong : Patients' Reaction", ODA News Review (An Overseas Doctors' Association Review), Vol.3, Issue No.12 (March-April), p.11.

95. The Times of India has introduced the system of ombudsman. It appointed Justice P.N. Bhagwati, retired chief Justice of India, as the ombudsman.

96. Havard, John (1992), " 'No fault' Compensation for Medical Accident", Medical Science Law, Vol. 32, No.3, p.187-197.

97. Grover, N.K. (1998), "Doctor-Patient Relationship : Today" Karol Bagh, Medical Society (KBMS) Newsletter, October.

98. Harvard, John (1992), op cit.

99. Ibid.

100. Ibid.

101. Indian Medical Association, (1993) Consumer Protection Act vis-à-vis Medical Profession, Indian Medical Association (IMA's)

Policy Document (New Delhi-IMA House).

102. Singh, Puspa and Hem Chandra (1998), 'Citizens' Charter versus Medical Ethics and Health legislation", Journal of the Indian Medical Association (JIMA),Vol.96, No.9 (September), p.282.

103. Ibid.

104. Grover, N. K. (1998), "Doctor-Patient Relationship Today", KBMS Newsletter, October.

105. Grover, N.K.(1992), Consumer Protection Act: IMA's View Point, Souvenir (National Seminar on the Problems of Medical Profession organised by Moradabad Branch of IMA on Sep. 13, 1992).

106. Ibid.

107. Grover, N.K. (1998), "Doctor-Patient Relationship Today", KBMS News Letter, October.

108. Ibid.

109. Jain, Kalpana (1995) "Malpractice Cases will Speed Up", The Hindustan Times, November, 28.

110. Grover N.K. (1992), op cit.

111. Ibid.

Chapter 2

Studies on Medical Services: Global and Indian Experiences

The objective of this chapter is to provide a brief account of the literature on the subject of patients' perception of medical services and their awareness about the Consumer Protection Act, 1986. All the studies conducted on the subject have been classified under two categories: (1) Studies conducted outside India. and (2) Studies conducted in India.

2.1 Studies Conducted Outside India

The studies conducted outside India, based on patients' perception of medical services, quality of patient-care, patient satisfaction, factors influencing physician's choice, patients' complaining behaviour and the practice of defensive medicines used by the doctors are briefly summarised below:

2.1.1 Studies Based on Patients' Perception: Taylor, et al. (1981) [1] felt that consumer opinion can yield valuable information about the functioning of health care system and that should be taken into account while assessing the quality of medical services provided. This study was conducted, through a survey, to assess the patients' perception of the quality of care. It was found that the performance of the hospital workers as assessed by the patients could be positively associated with the patients' satisfaction.

Casarreal, et al. (1986) [2] found that the process of implementing a multi-hospital monitoring system was delicate, requiring tact, diplomacy and willing participation by all administrators. They conducted the survey through a questionnaire. In the study, patients' perception was described as the degree to which patients ratings approached complete satisfaction with the services and attitude of the staff group. It was found that nursing services and attitudes, along with physician's attitude, were the most important determinants in evaluation of the behaviour of their staff and experience of the patients' with stay in the hospital. It was suggested that management could use the research data based on patients' perception to know which areas needed strengthening or correction.

Boscarino (1992) [3] analysed the overall quality rating of medical and surgical hospitals by type, size, staff ratio, mortality rate, case mix and their location. It was concluded that patients' survey data could be used to evaluate the quality of hospital care. Regardless of the method used to monitor quality, it was observed that the provision of quality care was an ongoing process.

2.1.2 Studies on Quality of Patient Care: Rhee (1976) [4] through a survey tried to find out the effects of physician's specialisation, type of medical school attended, experience, ambulatory care provided and the type of hospital on the quality of physician's performance in patients' care. The study indicated that the quality of care was influenced by physician's education, training and experience on the one hand, and the organisation of the setting in which care was provided, on the other hand.

In a survey [5] conducted in 1993 in New York city on 250 respondents who had been hospitalised overnight at least once during the preceding two years, it was found that about one-third of them were less than highly satisfied with the way their doctor explained their medical problem, treatment options and responded to their questions. Nearly the same number wanted better information about their clinical progress and what care they should take after discharge. Twenty percent of the respondents felt that they were given too little information about the anesthesia to be used and 10 percent felt that the surgeon did not inform them adequately about the procedure and its risks. Furthermore, one-third responded that nurses did not answer their queries or attend to their pain promptly.

Another survey [6] conducted in 1995 in New York City on 70,000 respondents on problems in the examination room, revealed that the medical care was far from ideal. It was found that 20 percent of doctors did not encourage questions and 29 percent of the doctors did not solicit patients' opinion about their condition. Most alarming, 26 percent failed to warn patients about the potential side-effects of the drugs they prescribed. It was concluded that patients were more likely to be satisfied overall with the doctor who encouraged questions, explained the side-effects of medication and made them feel at ease.

2.1.3 Studies on Patients' Satisfaction: Inguanzo (1985) [7] carried out a study to determine the level of patients' satisfaction with five factors relating to hospital stay: nursing care, appearance of the room, attitude of the hospital staff, quality of the food and billing procedures. It was found that perception of non-medical factors played a substantial role in the patient's overall evaluation of his hospital stay, though quality of medical care was the prime concern of hospital. It was suggested that every hospital should implement a mechanism to obtain reliable feedback from patients regarding various aspects of their stay and in the areas where there was substantial patients' dissatisfaction efforts should be made to determine the reasons for dissatisfaction and programme be set up to eliminate dissatisfaction.

Ross' study (1985) [8] revealed that even in the days of high consumer consciousness, the patients would reasonably complain if they were made to sit for hours in an out-patient department waiting for an appointment. The reasons for not making complaints were found to be the feeling of inevitability and irrational fear that complaining would lead to lesser care and treatment.

Heffring (1986) [9] surveyed 1300 patients discharged from the hospitals in the previous year for empirically measuring their level of satisfaction during their stay in the hospital. The study revealed that 'being treated as an individual' and 'having timely and adequate information about my condition' were more important to patient's satisfaction than the medical outcomes. The study also indicated that patients wanted to be more actively involved in the decision-making process concerning their care and treatment. The study concluded that the feedback generated by the study offered hospitals a marketing tool and a valuable opportunity to work together with patients to provide the best healthcare possible at the least cost.

Boscarino (1988) [10] analysed the hospital's ratings for 65 (non-government) hospitals across the United States. Over 14,000 customers were surveyed. The public's ratings of those local hospitals were analysed in terms of hospital size (number of beds), in-patient census, the urbanity level of local areas, and the level of care provided. A multivariate analysis of the data indicated that hospital ratings were significantly related to the level of care provided and the hospital size. The study revealed that consumers rated and chose hospitals based on the characteristics of facilities provided. Further, it was found that more affluent consumers were more discriminating and that the hospitals that provided a higher level of care, were located in more metropolitan areas. The study suggested that a hospital's perceived quality was important and could affect admissions.

2.1.4 Studies on Factors Influencing Physician's Choice: Hill (1991) [11] interviewed 205 adults and investigated the importance of criteria in their final choice of a physician. The study showed that the criteria directly related to the physician's understanding of the patients' medical needs and competence in taking care of those problems were of primary importance in the choice of a physician. The criteria included were : 'seems knowledgeable', 'seems interested in my problem', 'explains what is being done and why', 'offers practical solutions to my problems', 'asks appropriate questions about my problem', and 'spends enough time with me'. The study found that the next three highest ranked criteria were related to increasing the patients' comfort, which included 'treat me in a personal manner', 'hire competent assistants', and 'is not pushy or abrasive in manner'. The study suggested that knowledge of patient's choice criteria was of direct value to the physicians in private or group practice as a means of building and maintaining a client base in a very competitive market place.

2.1.5 Study on Patients' Complaining Behaviour: Dolinsky (1995) [12] through a survey of 472 elderly and near-elderly persons found that 17 percent of respondents (typically in the last 2 years) made complaint about some aspects of their visit to physician's office. The analysis revealed five underlying dimensions that reflected their satisfaction or dissatisfaction with health care services received while visiting a physician, namely, the quality of physician, the quality of nurses, the quality of administrative personnel, the cost of health care and access to health care. Dolinsky suggested that health care providers must ensure that they possessed the appropriate complaint information and they should establish in-house mechanism to solicit and resolve complaints, something akin to customer service group or ombudsman found in many organisations.

2.1.6 Studies on Practice of Defensive Medicine: Practice of using defensive medicine by doctors implies ordering every possible laboratory test, X-ray, scan and second opinion by doctors solely to protect themselves from the future claims of negligence.

Defensive medicine consists of 'adopting procedures which are not for the benefit of the patient but safeguard against the possibility of the patient making a claim for negligence [*White House vs. Jordan* (1980), 1 All ER 650, 659].

In a study conducted by Pollack (1980) [13] through a survey of 4020 practising physicians, of whom 35 percent responded, the practising physicians were asked whether concern about legal liability had led them to make any of 15 specific practice changes. It was found that over 80 percent doctors checked at least one option. The result indicated that 48 percent doctors ordered more tests to avoid risks, 44 percent maintained more detailed patients' records, 40 percent used more consultations, 30 percent stopped performing certain procedures, 25 percent accepted new patients more selectively, 24 percent scheduled more follow-up visits, 20 percent used consent forms for more procedures, 18 percent hospitalised more cases, 17 percent stuck closer to recommended drug dosages, 16 percent took more extensive initial histories and 14 percent delegated fewer medical procedures. In this study only 30 percent of the respondents were subjected to threats of suits and only 20 percent had formal claims filed against them and only 10 percent had been in litigation.

In a study conducted through a survey in 1984, by American College of Surgeons [14], it has been reported that doctors often stopped performing certain procedures or stopped practising in a particular area of specialisation for reasons associated with malpractice litigation. It was found that 40 percent doctors were no longer accepting high risk cases in consultations and 28 percent were not performing certain procedures solely because of risks of malpractice suits.

Gleicner (1984) [15] expressed the view that the defensive practices entailed more than just ordering extra tests. He observed that obstetricians in the US were performing caesarean sections at a rate much higher than that anywhere in the world. However, he expressed that clear definition of defensive practice, its nature and reliable estimates of its extent were difficult to find.

Reynolds (1987) [16] found that the cost of unnecessary medical practices was difficult to estimate and might vary from 15 percent of the total expenditure for physicians services to 30 percent of the total cost of healthcare.

Quam, et al. (1987) [17] in their study reported that 40 percent of physicians admitted ordering additional tests and 27 percent carried out additional procedures as a response to the fear of litigation. They stated that it added 5 percent to the total US healthcare expenditure. The same survey reported an appreciable improvement in record-keeping because of the fear of litigation.

2.2 Studies Conducted in India

A summary of the studies conducted in India on patients' satisfaction, consumers' awareness of the Consumer Protection Act, 1986, its benefits to consumers and the professional indemnity insurance taken up by the doctors, is presented below :

2.2.1 Studies Based on Patients' Satisfaction: Timmappaya, et al. (1971) [18] in their study tried to assess the patients' satisfaction through a survey conducted in two hospitals of Delhi. The findings of the study showed that patients' satisfaction was associated with the educational level of the patients. It also showed that longer stay in the hospital resulted in higher satisfaction rate. Factors like food, non-communication of diagnosis, discharge policy and behaviour of sweepers contributed to dissatisfaction of the patients.

Another study carried out by Timmappaya, et al. [19] in 1973 in five general hospitals in Delhi, revealed that the points of satisfaction of the patients were the behaviour of the doctors and nurses on duty and their line of treatment. The points of patients' dissatisfaction were non-communication of diagnosis, sanitary conditions, behaviour of hospital staff and influence of out-patient waiting facilities.

Nath (1973) [20] conducted a study about the health needs, expectations and satisfaction of the CGHS beneficiaries in Delhi. The study, based on interview of 184 patients, revealed that while 80 percent of the patients were satisfied with the services provided to them, only one-third were satisfied with the time spent on them by the doctor. Further, it was found that nearly 60 percent of the patients were satisfied with the medicine prescribed.

Mitra (1975) [21] sought to evaluate the quality of in-patient services in a district hospital in Haryana. He laid more stress on indirect measures such as promptness in carrying out the investigation, which in the long run, invariably improved the quality of care. It was suggested in the study that doctors should see every patient at least once in a day and nursing staff should take more interest in attending to the patients after their admission. Percentage of errors in pulse checking, rate of doctor's round and percentage of essential therapies not administered to patients can be used as indicators to judge the quality of care. It was concluded that improvements in these variables was likely to enhance the overall quality of medical care in the hospital.

Bhatnagar (1985) [22] conducted a study to determine the patients' satisfaction with Employee's State Insurance (ESI) scheme in Rajasthan. A total of 190 patients were interviewed through a questionnaire. Findings of the study revealed that the good behaviour of the doctor and of the para-medical staff contributed to satisfaction of majority of patients. But three-fourth of the patients expressed their dissatisfaction with the organisation of out-patient services, involving long waiting time and quality of drugs supplied to them.

Satia (1986) [23] tried to assess the patients' satisfaction in ESI dispensaries, through a survey of 202 patients. The results showed that the majority of the patients were satisfied. The patients who were dissatisfied gave reasons such as 'doctors did not examine properly', 'medicines were not good', 'it took a lot of time to get services' and 'had to come to the dispensary too often'.

2.2.2 Study on CPA's Benefits to Consumers: Singh(1990) [24] undertook a study through a sample of 105 consumers in Delhi, to find out their attitude towards various business marketing activities and the role played by manufacturers and the government in protecting the interest of consumers. It was found that an overwhelming majority (85 percent) of the respondents felt that most of the manufacturers were more interested in making profits than in satisfying the consumers. Almost all felt that if a consumer got injured or fell ill while using a product, which was defective, the manufacturer should pay the damages, indicating that the consumers had the feeling that the manufacturer should be held liable for the quality of their products or services.

It was also reported in the study that over 76 percent of the respondents felt that from their point of view the procedure followed by most manufacturers and government in handling complaints and settling grievances was not satisfactory. While, 79 percent attributed this sorry state of affairs to lack of consumer education, 80 percent felt that the CPA would be helpful in protecting and promoting the interests of the consumers. An overwhelming majority (86 percent) of consumers also believed that the average person was willing to pay higher price for quality product that would ensure health and safety standards.

2.2.3 Studies on Consumers' Awareness of CPA: In a study [25], conducted in 1995 by the Indian Institute of Public Administration (IIPA), sponsored by the Ministry of Civil Supplies, Consumer Affairs and Public Distribution, of the Government of India, in 10 districts covering five States, it was found that out of 1168 persons who were approached, 976 (83.56 percent) were unaware of the consumer protection measures contained in the Consumer Protection Act and 1051 persons (89.91 percent) did not know how to file a complaint in the Consumer Court.

Sawarkar (1996) [26] undertook a study in Marathwada. The survey was conducted on 750 respondents selected randomly during 1994 and 1995. It was found that majority of the respondents (51.33 percent) were totally ignorant of the consumer protection measures contained in the CPA, 1986, and 49.12 percent of the respondents were unaware of redressal machinery established under the Act and still, more number of respondents (54.38 percent) were not even aware of complaint lodging procedure. It was also revealed that 36.84 percent respondents did not insist on a purchase receipt. It was found that lack of awareness and absence of documents of purchase were the main reasons for not lodging complaints by consumers for their dissatisfaction. It was suggested that education programmes for creating awareness about the CPA should be arranged by voluntary consumer organisations, the government and other social welfare institutions.

2.2.4 Study on Professional Indemnity Insurance: Random inquiries made by the Indian Express News Service [27] at private nursing homes in various parts of the capital revealed that a majority of the practising doctors had either already acquired a policy of professional indemnity insurance or were planning to soon acquire one. Even those who were already insured had decided to hike the amount of their insurance cover.

2.3 Conclusion

From the above studies it appears that medical care is still far from what patients expected as ideal. The main reasons indicated by these studies include : non-communication on the part of doctors, behavioural attitude of staff and delay in treatment. It has also been revealed by these studies that consumer awareness, though presently less, is on the increase in India. Review of the studies conducted abroad has revealed that patients wanted to be involved in the decision-making process about their care and treatment. Further, these studies indicated that it was the fear of litigation and payment of huge compensation that compelled doctors to indulge in defensive medical practices. Basically, these steps were seemingly resorted to by medical professional just to protect themselves. However, on the positive side, it has also been found that doctors were becoming more careful and they took interest in writing elaborate patients' records, tried to give more information to the patients and involved them in the treatment process. However, there has been a lack of Indian studies on this subject and no major study has so far been conducted either by the government or by the management of private health institutions to assess the patients' perception of medical services, their awareness of the CPA as a means of redressal of their grievances and to examine the impact of application of the CPA to medical services on the patient-doctor relationship. The topic appeared to be under-researched in India.

It was felt that a more comprehensive study on the subject of CPA and medical negligence was required. Accordingly, the present study has been undertaken in order to bridge this gap.

Notes

1. Taylor, P.W., Nelson, E., et al. (1981), "Development and Use of a Method of Assessing Patients' Perception of Care", Hospital and Health Services Administration, Winter, pp.89-104.

2. Casarreal, Kenia, M., et al. (1986), "Improving Service through Patients' Survey in a Multi-Hospital Organisation", Hospital and Health Services Administration, Vol. 31, No.2 (March-April), pp.41-49.

3. Boscarino, Joseph A. (1992), "The Public's Perception of Quality Hospital : Implications of Patients' Surveys", Hospital and Health Services Administration, Spring, pp. 13-35.

4. Rhee, Sang-O (1976), "Factors Determining the Quality of Physician's Performance in Patient Care", Medical Care, Vol. 14, No. 9 (September), pp. 733-750.

5. Consumers Report (1995), "How is Your Doctor Treating You ?", Vol.16, No.2 (February), pp. 81-86.

6. Ibid.

7. Inguanzo, Joe, M. and Mark Harju (1985), "Consumer's Satisfaction with Hospitalisation", Hospitals, May 1, pp. 81-84.

8. Ross, H.R. (1985), "Customer Service in a Hospital Out-Patient Department", Hospital and Health Services Review, November, pp. 274-277.

9. Heffring , Michael, P., et al. (1986), "High Tech, High Touch: Common Denomination in Patient Satisfaction", Hospital and Health Services Administration , March-April, pp. 81-94.

10. Boscarino, Joseph A. (1988), "The Public's Rating of Hospitals", Hospital and Health Services Administration, Vol. 33, No. 2, (Summer), pp. 189-198.

11. Hill, Jeanne, C. (1991), "Factors Influencing Physician's Choice", Hospital and Health Services Administration, Winter, pp. 491-503.

12. Dolinsky, Arthur L. (1995), "Complaint Intensity and Health Care Services" Journal of Health Care Marketing (A Journal of American Marketing Association), Vol. 15 (Summer), pp. 42-47.

13. Pollack, R.S. (1980), Clinical Aspects of Malpractice (New Jersey : Medical Economics Company, Book Division).

14. Professional Liability Survey Report (1984), Chicago : American College of Surgeons, as cited in "Professional Liability : No Fault Solution", New England Journal of Medicine (1990), Vol. 332, No.9, pp. 627-631.

15. Gleicner, N. (1984), "Cesarean Section Rates in United States: The Short Term Failure of the National Consensus Development Conference in 1980", Journal of American Medical Association (JAMA), Vol.2, No.52, pp. 3273 - 6.

16. Reynolds, R.A., J.A. Rizzo and M.L. Gongalez (1987), "The Cost of Medical Professional Liability", Journal of American Medical Association (JAMA), Vol. 252, pp. 2776-81.

17. Quam, L., R. Dingwall and P. Fenn (1987), "Medical Malpractice in Perspective : The American Experience", British Medical Journal , June, pp. 1529-1531.

18. Timmappaya, A. and Aggarwal, et al. (1971), Patients' Satisfaction and Ward Social System, National Institute of Health and Family Welfare, Research Report No. 3, New Delhi.

19. Timmappaya, A., S. Chatopadhaya, K.G. Agarwal and M. Advani (1973), Hospital and its People, National Institute of Health and Family Welfare, Research Report No. 15, New Delhi.

20. Nath, N.A. (1973), unpublished M.D. thesis, entitled "A Study of Central Government Health Scheme in Relation to Health Needs" in Faculty of Medical Sciences, National Institute of Health and Family Welfare, University of Delhi, New Delhi.

21. Mitra, S. K. (1975), unpublished thesis, entitled "Evaluation of In-patient Services in District Hospital", in National Institute of Health and Family Welfare, New Delhi.

22. Bhatnagar, Deepak (1985), Labour Welfare and Social Security Legislation in India (New Delhi : Deep and Deep Publications).

23. Satia, Harish Kumar (1986), unpublished thesis, entitled "A Study of the Factors affecting the Out- Patient Care as well as Effective Working of the Functional Dispensaries under ESI in Delhi" in National Institute of Health and Family Welfare, New Delhi.

24. Singh, R. (1990), "Consumers' Attitude towards Consumerism: An Exploratory Study", Consumer Confrontation, Vol. 10, No. 1, pp. 8-11.

25. As cited in Mathew, N.M. (1995), "Consumer Movement in India at Crossroads", Health for the Millions, October, p. 75.

26. Sawarkar, J.G. (1996), "Consumer Awareness : A Survey Analysis" Indian Journal of Marketing, No. 10-11-12, Vol. 25 (October), pp. 13-21.

27. Express News Service (1995), "Supreme Court Order Drives Doctors to Seek Insurance Cover", Indian Express, November, 16.

Chapter 3

Medical Services in India: Regulatory Measures

This chapter seeks to briefly analyse the legal measures for redressal of patients complaints, including the relevant provisions of the Consumer Protection Act, 1986. Major cases decided under the CPA, 1986, by the National Commission and various State Commissions in India, relating to deficiency in medical services since their inception till January 31, 2001, are also reviewed in order to evaluate the approach of the Consumer Courts in deciding such cases.

Various laws have been enacted to provide safety to patients by regulating medical practices in India. Apart from the Consumer Protection Act, 1986, there are some other laws, which are applicable to the medical profession. The major provisions of the legislations under which a patient can seek redressal of their grievances against deficiency and negligence in the provision of the medical services are briefly analysed below.

3.1 Relevant Provisions of the Indian Contract Act, 1872

Under the Indian Contract Act, 1872, when a patient goes to a doctor for medical treatment, he enters into an implied contract with him, that the doctor will use reasonable professional skill and care. If the doctor fails to fulfil his contractual obligation in the performance of contract, i.e. if the medical treatment is found injurious to the patient, the patient can take action under Section 73 of the Indian Contract Act, 1872, for breach of contract in a Civil Court but he will have to pay a prescribed court fee as specified by the Court Fee Act, 1870, according to the amount being claimed by him. This course of action is not popular with patients because the suit can only be filed in the Civil Court where an advocate will have to be engaged and the court fee will have to be paid before filing the suit.

3.2 Provisions of the Indian Penal Code, 1860

In case of death due to negligence, the doctor can be sued under Section 304-A of the Indian Penal Code (IPC). In case of injuries lesser than death, the remedy is available under Section 336,337 and 338 of the IPC.

Section 304A: Causing Death by Negligence: Whosoever causes the death of any person by doing any rash or negligent act not amounting to culpable homicide, shall be punished with imprisonment of either description for a term which may extend to two years, or with fine, or with both [1].

Section 304-A of the Indian Penal Code carves out a specific offence where death is caused by doing a rash or negligent act and that act does not amount to culpable homicide or murder. Doing an act with the intent to kill a person or knowledge that doing of an act was likely to cause a persons death are ingredient of an offence of culpable homicide, thus, the provision of the Section 304-A apply to cases where there is no intention to cause death and no knowledge that the act done in all probability would cause death. It only applies to cases in which, without any such intention or knowledge, death is caused by a rash or negligent act.

Section 336: Act endangering life or personal safety of others: Whoever does any act so rashly or negligently as to endanger human life or the personal safety of others shall be punishable with imprisonment of either description for a term which may extend to three months, or with fine which may extend to two hundred fifty rupees, or with both [2].

Section 337: Causing hurt by act endangering life or personal safety of others: Whoever causes hurt to any person by doing any act so rashly or negligently as to endanger human life, or the personal safety of others, shall be punished with imprisonment of either description for a term which may extend to six months, or with fine which may extend to five hundred rupees, on with both [3].The offence punishable under Section 337 is an aggravated form of offence under Section 336.

Section 338: Causing grievous hurt by act endangering life or personal safety of others: Whoever causes grievous hurt to any person by doing any act so rashly or negligently as to endanger human life, or the personal safety of others, shall be punished with imprisonment of either description for a term which may extend to two years, or with fine which may extend to one thousand rupees, or with both [4].

Mere negligence or rashness is not enough to bring a case within the ambit of Section 337 or Section 338 of IPC. Negligence or rashness proved by evidence must be such as should carry with it a criminal liability.

Thus, if a patient or his guardian or heir has any complaint of negligent act on the part of a doctor, he can lodge a complaint with the police, under Sections 304-A, 336,337 and 338 of the Indian Penal Code. On receipt of the complaint, the police is empowered to make investigations in the matter and if there is any substance in the complaint, it can register a case and try it in a Criminal Court. If the complainant is able to prove the negligence on the part of the doctor, the doctor can be punished with imprisonment or fine or both, according to the gravity of the negligence and punishment prescribed under the Indian Penal Code. Unfortunately in India, patients and their attendants often afraid of approaching the police, for the police here are not looked upon as friends of the people as in UK but as, adversaries. Hence, a criminal complaint is hardly ever registered under the Indian Penal Code.

3.3 Relevant Provisions of the Law of Torts

An aggrieved patient can file a suit in the Civil Courts under the Law of Torts to claim damages. Negligence is a tort, i.e., a wrong done by one person to another. In medical terms, it has been defined as a mistake by a doctor which no reasonable, competent and careful doctor should have committed.

According to this law, negligence is both a civil and a criminal wrong. As a civil wrong, it has been defined as a breach of legal duty to take care to prevent damages, loss or injury.

Thus, if a doctor does not take the degree of care which he is required to take and causes injury to his patient, the patient can sue him under the Law of Torts. He can claim damages but he will have to pay the court fee according to the amount claimed and will have to engage an advocate to pursue his suit. Not many suits are filed under the Law of Torts because it takes a long time to decide such cases. Both these factors dissuade people from pursuing this legal remedy.

3.4 Relevant Provisions of the Indian Medical Council Act, 1956

A complaint can be lodged with the State Medical Council which is authorised to suspend or even terminate registration of negligent doctor.

The Indian Medical Council Act (IMC Act) came into force in 1956. The Act confers powers to the Medical Council of India to discipline erring members of the medical profession. However, this Act does not have any provision for the award of damages to the complainant, though it has enough powers to punish the medical practitioners. The Council is empowered to take disciplinary action against doctors committing professional misconduct. Section 24 empowers the Council to direct the removal of name of any person enrolled on a state medical register on the grounds of professional misconduct.

The IMC Act also confers powers on the Council to prescribe standards of professional conduct and etiquette and code of ethics for medical practitioners. The State Medical Councils investigate complaints of professional misconduct. The Medical Councils can themselves initiate inquiry against a doctor for misconduct or they may do so when a complaint is received from anyone regarding such misconduct of the doctor. Such complaint must be in writing, signed by the complainant and should have all the relevant facts.

A doctor has to keep himself abreast of new and fresh

discoveries in the medical sciences, which means be cannot rest contended with what he had learnt in his students days. The Medical Councils, which are supposed to self-regulate the medical profession by monitoring their skills and conduct, are doing almost nothing to provide continuous education and disciplining of the doctors who resort to unethical practices [5].

The data given in a study [6] suggest that even in developed countries about one out of ten independently functioning doctors is found to be deficient and to an extent, incompetent in providing reasonable quality care.

The National Commission in *Cosmopolitan Hospital v. Vasantha P. Nair* observed [7]:

"There is no provision in the Indian Medical Council Act, 1956 for the protection of the interest of the persons who have suffered on account of negligence or deficiency in the services rendered by medical profession. The field left open by the said Act is covered by the law of Torts in general and by the Consumer Protection Act in particular."

3.5 The Consumer Protection Act, 1986 and Medical Services

The Consumer Protection Act (CPA), 1986 was passed by the Indian Parliament in December 1986 [8]. The first amendment in the Act came into force on June 15, 1991 and further the Act was amended by the Consumer Protection (Amendment) Ordinance, 1993 (No.24 of 1993) dated June 18, 1993 [9] which subsequently was passed by the Rajya Sabha on August 5, 1993 and the Lok Sabha on August 20, 1993 and was assented to by the President of India on August 27, 1993. However, the Amendment Act was deemed to have come into force with effect from June 18, 1993.

The Consumer Protection Bill 1986

It was introduced in the Parliament with the following statement of objects and reasons:

1. The Bill seeks to provide for better protection of interest of

consumers and for that purpose, to make provisions for the establishment of consumer councils and other authorities, for the settlement of consumers disputes and for matters connected therewith.

2. It seeks, interalia, to promote and protect the right of consumers such as

a. The right to be protected against marketing of goods which are hazardous to life and property.

b. The right to be informed about the quality, quantity, potency, purity, standard and price of goods to protect the consumer against unfair trade practices.

c. The right to be assured, wherever possible, access to variety of goods at competitive price.

d. The right to be heard and to be assured that consumer interest will receive due consideration at appropriate forums.

e. The right to seek redressal against unfair trade practice or unscrupulous exploitation of consumers; and

f. Right to consumer education.

3. These objects are sought to be promoted and protected by the Consumer Protection Council to be established at the Central and State level.

4. To provide speedy and simple redressal to consumer disputes, a quasi-judicial machinery is sought to be set up at the District, State and Central level. These quasi-judicial bodies will observe the principles of natural justice and have been empowered to give relief of a specific nature and to award, wherever appropriate, compensation to consumer. Penalties for non-compliance of the orders given by the quasi-judicial bodies have also been provided.

The Consumer Protection (Amendment) Bill 1991

It was introduced in the Parliament with the following statement of objects and reasons:

In view of the recent decision of the National Consumer Dispute Redressal Commission (National Commission) regarding the order under sub section 2 of Section 14 of the Act, it was felt that the said Act required certain modifications. Accordingly, the Consumer Protection (Amendment) Ordinance 1991 was promulgated to provide interalia:

a. For amendment of sub-section 2 of section 14 to provide that every proceeding of the District Forum shall be conducted by the President and at least one member thereof sitting together.

b. That every order made by the District Forum shall be signed by its President and member or members who conducted the proceedings.

The Consumer Protection (Amendment) Bill 1993

It was introduced in the Parliament with the following statements of objects and reasons:

In the year 1986, the Consumer Protection Act was enacted to provide the better protection of interest of Consumers and for that purpose to make provisions for the establishment of consumer councils and other authorities for the settlement of consumer disputes and matter connected therewith. The working of redressal agencies set up under the Act has helped to raise the expectations of the people and also brought to the focus certain inadequacies in the coverage of the Act. The Consumer Protection (Amendment) Bill 1993 seeks to plug these loopholes and enlarge the scope of areas covered and entrust more powers to the redressal agencies under the Act. Accordingly, the Bill interalia, seeks to provide for followings:

a. To enlarge the scope of the Act so as to enable the consumers to file class action complaints where such consumers have a common interest and to file complaints relating to restrictive trade practices adopted by a trader.

b. To enable the consumers who are self-employed to file complaints before the redressal agencies where goods bought by them exclusively for earning their livelihood, suffer from any defect.

c. To add 'services' relating to housing constructions.

d. To enable filing of class action complaints on behalf of group of consumers having the same interest.

e. To provide for the constitution of selection committees for the selection of non-judicial members of various redressal agencies.

f. To increase the monetary jurisdiction of District Fora/State Commission/National Commission.

g. To confer additional powers on the redressal agencies by way of awarding cost of the parties for ordering removal of defects or deficiency from the services and for empowering to recall of goods likely to endanger the safety of public etc.

h. To impose punishment on the complaint in cases of frivolous or vexatious complaints; and

i. To provide a limitation period of one year for filing complaints.

The aims and objects of the Act, interalia, are : better protection of the interest of consumers and speedy settlement of disputes as against civil actions, which are costly and time consuming. Provisions of the Act are in addition to, and not in derogation of, any other law for time being in force and are compulsory in nature.

The Act postulates the establishment of Central Consumer Protection Council and State Consumer Protection Council and the objects of both these councils are one and the same viz., the rights to be protected against marketing of goods and services which are hazardous to life and property, the right to be informed about the quality, quantity, potency, purity, standard and price of goods or services as the case may be so as to protect the consumer against unfair trade practices, the right to be assured wherever possible access to a variety of goods and services at competitive prices; the right to be heard and to be assured that consumers' interest will receive due consideration at appropriate forums; the right to seek redressal against unfair trade practices or restrictive trade practices or unscrupulous exploitation of consumers and the right to consumer education [10].

No court fee or stamp duty is required to be paid as against the existing procedure in all judicial forums in India. An individual can himself plead his case or he can take assistance of a registered consumer group or society or organisation. Presence of advocates to plead the case is not essential.

The machinery created under the Act endeavours to provide speedy, simple and inexpensive redressal of the grievances of consumers ranging from defective household appliances to medical services. The Consumer Protection Act is mainly compensation-oriented. Thus, any patient who has any grievance against a doctor or health institution can approach the forums of the CPA to seek redressal of his complaint.

3.5.1 Relevant Terms

Section 2(1) of the Act provides the definition of the various terms used in the Act. Some important definitions having a bearing on its applications to services rendered by medical profession are as follows :

Complainant: According to Section 2(1) (b), Complainant means (i) a consumer; or (ii) any voluntary consumer association registered under the Companies Act, 1956 or under any other law for the time being in force ; or (iii) the Central Government or any State Government, who or which makes a complaint; or (iv) one or more consumers, where there are numerous consumers having the same interest [11].

Complaint: According to Section 2(1) (c), Complaint means any allegation in writing made by a complainant that : (i) an unfair trade practice or a restrictive trade practice has been adopted by any trader; (ii) the goods bought by him or agreed to be bought by him suffer from one or more defects, (iii) the services hired or availed of or agreed to be hired or availed of by him [12] suffer from deficiency in any respect with a view to obtain any relief provided by or under this Act, (iv) a trader has charged for the goods mentioned in the complaint a price in excess of the price fixed by or under any law for the time being in force or displayed on the goods of any package containing such goods, (v) goods which will be hazardous to life and safety when used, are being offered for sale to the public in contravention of the provisions of any law for the time being in force requiring traders to display information in regard to the contents, manner and effect of use of such goods.

Thus, complaint is a statement made in writing to the National Commission, the State Commission or the District Forum by a person competent to file it, containing the allegations in details, and with a view to obtain relief provided under the Act.

The 'Unfair Trade Practice' means - a trade practice which, for the purpose of promoting the sale, use or supply of any goods or for the provision of any service, adopts any unfair methods or unfair or deceptive practice including any of the following practices, namely:

1. The practice of making any statement whether orally or in writing or by visible representation which, falsely represents;

a. that the goods are of a particular standard, quality, quantity, grade, composition, style or model;

b. any re-built, second-hand, renovated, reconditioned or old goods as new goods.

c. the services are of a particular standard, quality or grade.

d. the goods or services have sponsorship, approval, performance, characteristics, accessories, uses or benefits which such goods or services do not have.

e. the seller or the supplier has a sponsorship or approval or affiliation which such seller or supplier does not have.

f. concerning the need for, or the usefulness of any goods or services.

g. gives to the public any warranty or guarantee of the performance, efficacy or length of life of a product o of any goods that is not based on an adequate or proper test thereof;

h. makes to the public a representation in a form that purports to be a warranty or guarantee of a product or of any goods of services, or a promise to replace, maintain or repair an article or any part thereof or to repeat or continue a service until it has achieved a specified result, if such purported warranty or guarantee or promise is materially misleading or if there is no reasonable prospect that such warranty, guarantee or promise will be carried out.

i. materially misleads the public concerning the price at which a product or like products or goods or services, have been or are, ordinarily sold or provided, and, for this purpose, a representation as to price shall be deemed to refer to the price at which the product or goods or services has or have been sold by sellers or provided by suppliers generally in the relevant market unless it is clearly specified to be the price at which the product has been sold or services have been provided by the person by whom or on whose behalf the representation is made.

j. disparaging the goods, services or trade of another person.

2. Permits the publication of any advertisement whether in any newspaper or otherwise, for the sale or supply at a bargain price, of goods or services that are not intended to be offered the sale of supply at the bargain price, or for a period that is, and in quantities that are, reasonable, having regard to the nature of the market in which the business is carried on, the nature and size of business, and the nature of the advertisement.

3. Permits the offering of gifts, prizes or other items with the intention of not providing them as offered or creating impression that something is being given or offered free of charge when it is fully or partly covered by the amount charged in the transaction as a whole; or the conduct of any contest, lottery, game of chance or skill, for the purpose of promoting, directly or indirectly, the sale, use or supply of any product or any business interest.

4. Permits the sale or supply of goods intended to be used, or are of a kind likely to be used, by consumer, knowing or having reason to believe that the goods do not comply with the standards prescribed by competent authority relating to performance, composition, contents, design, constructions, finishing or packaging as are necessary to prevent or reduce the risk of injury to the person using the goods.

5. Permits the hoping or destruction of goods, or refuses to sell the goods or to make them available for sale or to provide

any service, if such hoarding or destruction or refusal raised or tends to raise or is intended to raise, the cost of those or other similar goods or services.

The 'restrictive trade practice' means the trade practice which requires a consumer to buy, hire or avail of any goods, or, as the case may be, services as a condition precedent for buying, hiring or availing of other goods or services.

Complaint Can Be Filed by

The consumer himself or

Beneficiary of the consumer: A consumer is not only the person who hires or avails any service for consideration but also the person who is beneficiary of services. (*K. B. Jayalaxmi vs. Govt of Tamil Nadu and Ors.* 1994 (1) CPR 114).

LR of the deceased consumer: There are no express words indicating that the legal representatives of a consumer are also included within its scope but by operation of law, the legal representatives get clothed with the rights and status. (*Cosmopolitan Hospital and Anr. vs. Smt. Vasantha P. Nair* (1) 1992 CPJ NC 302).

Legal Heirs of the deceased consumers: A legal heir of the deceased consumer can well maintain a complaint under the Act (*Joseph Alias Animon and Anr. vs. Dr. Elizabeth Zachariah and Ors* (1) 1997 CPJ 96).

Parents of a minor: Where a young child is taken to the hospital by his parents and the child is treated by the doctor, the parents of such a minor child can file the claim for compensation under the Act (*Spring Meadows Hospital and Anr. vs. Harjot Ahluwalia* JT 1998 (2) SC 620).

Husband of the consumer: In the Indian condition women may be illiterate, educated women may be unaware of their legal rights and to insist that the husband cannot file and prosecute complaints under the Consumer Protection Act on behalf of their spouses will deprive millions of consumers of the benefits of this legislation [13].

By a Relative: Smt. Smita Govilkar signed original complaint and merely because her father-in-law initiated the complaint, it cannot be said that it was a complaint by a non-consumer [14].

Registered Consumer Association

Society registered under MRTP Act.

Society Registered under the Societies Act: Mumbai Grahak Panchayat being a voluntary consumer organisation from Bombay registered under the Societies Act, 1860, is competent to be a complainant [15].

Insurance Company: Where Insurance Company is subrogated to rights of insured after settling and paying latter's claim, and insured executed a Special Power of Attorney and a letter of subrogation in favour of Insurance Company and thereby assigned transferred and subrogated all their rights against the defendant and authorise them to recover the amount in dispute from the defendant, it can file complaint for loss caused to the insured goods due to negligence of employees of the transport company [16].

Complaint Cannot be Filed

On behalf of the public which consists of unidentifiable consumers: In a case, the complaint was filed on behalf of unidentified number of purchasers of the biscuits of the opposite party, it was held that "the Scheme of the complaint consumers alone can receive the reliefs which may be granted under the Act. The public which consists of unidentifiable consumers cannot be granted the relief under the Act and as such to this extent the complaint does not conform to the provisions of the Act [17]."

By an individual for benefit of general public: The complainant being individual filed a complaint for the benefit of general public in a representative capacity. It was held that such a complaint could not be permitted [18].

Unregistered Association: The complainant was an association formed in the Gulf and was unregistered in India. It was held that since the petitioner is not a voluntary organisation registered under any law in force in India, the petitioner association being unregistered cannot come within clause (d) of

Section 2(1) and cannot file the complaint under the Act [19].

Complaint Must be Precise: The complaint was a jumbled and incoherent mass of facts and the complainant had failed to establish precisely how and in what respect the opposite party has failed to discharge its obligations to the complainant. It is not maintainable [20].

Subjudice - if the matter is pending in civil court : The subject matter of the complaint was subjudice in suits pending before the civil court and entertainment of the complaint was a clear overlapping and intervening of the questions arising for the determination in the suits, the appropriate forum is civil court and not the forum [21].

Subjudice - Not - if the matter is pending in criminal court: This commission has adopted, on its own, the rule of prudence that when a case is already subjudice, it will for bear to entertain a complaint under the Consumer Protection Act in the same case. Such a course of action is essential to avoid conflicting findings by different judicial and semi-judicial forums. It also obviates multiplicity of trial on the same cause of action. However, this is not true in this case, where the case is subjudice in a criminal court in as much as the relief obtainable and the parties which can obtain relief are entirely different. There is no question of granting relief as provided under Section 14 of the Consumer Protection Act, 1986 by the Metropolitan Magistrate. Consequently, it cannot be maintained by the State Commission on the ground that the case was subjudice being under investigation by the Metropolitan Magistrate [22].

Resjudicata

It is well settled principle of law that one cannot agitate same cause of action before a court of law of other adjudicating Forum after it has already been adjudicated upon earlier. This is the basis for the relevant provisions under the Civil Procedure Code (CPC) which embody a sound principle of law to obviate multiplicity of litigation. Even though the consumer forums are not governed by all the provisions of CPC, yet the sound principle of law and procedure embodied in the code are followed by the forums [23].

Consumer: The 'Consumer' as defined in *Blacks law dictionary* means, one who consumes. Individuals who purchase, use, maintain and dispose of product and services and users of final product are all included in the term consumer.

Consumer means any person who: (i) buys any goods for a consideration which has been paid or promised or partly paid and partly promised, or under any system of deferred payment and includes any user of such goods other than the person who buys such goods for consideration paid or promised or partly paid or partly promised, or under any system of deferred payment when such use is made with the approval of such person, but does not include a person who obtains such goods for re-sale or for any commercial purpose; or (ii) hires (or avails of) [24] any services for a consideration which has been paid or promised or partly paid and partly promised, or under any system of deferred payment and includes any beneficiary of such services other than the person who hires (or avails of) the services for consideration paid or promised, or partly paid and partly promised or under any system of deferred payment when such services are availed of with the approval of the first mentioned person.

Patient is a Consumer

The 'services' rendered by private medical practitioners and private nursing homes and hospitals, government hospitals, health centres and dispensaries, if not free are covered within the definition of 'services' and the person who avails the said services is a Consumer [25].

The activity of providing medical assistance for payment carried on by hospitals and members of medical profession falls within the scope of service as defined under Section 2(1) (o) of the Act and the persons who avails such services is a Consumer under the Act [26].

Consumer Includes Beneficiary

A consumer is not only the person who hires or avails any services for consideration but also the person who is beneficiary of such services [27].

Consumer Includes the legal representatives (LRs) of the Deceased Consumer

The legal representatives of the deceased consumer are also included as Consumer under the Act. In *Cosmopolitan Hospital & Anr. v. Vasantha P. Nair* [28], the National Commission observed, "In our opinion, it is consistent with the object and scheme of the Act and conductive for the achievement and promotion of the legislative purpose underlying the statute to give an extended meaning to the expression consumer defined in Section 2(1) (d) of the Act so as to include legal representative of deceased consumers."

Parents of minors as consumers

Parents of a minor are consumers within the meaning of the term consumer as defined in the Act. The definition of the term consumer is wide enough to include not only the person who hires the services but also the beneficiary of such services. Thus, both the parents of the child as well as the child would be consumer within the meaning of Section 2(1) (d) of the Act and they can claim compensation under the Act [29].

Any person who buys any goods or hires any services, in order to be called a consumer, must satisfy the following conditions.

(a) Buying of goods or hiring of services should be made against payment whether paid or promised to be paid or bought under deferred payment system; (b) goods or services should be bought for self use; and (c) the person using such goods or services, even though not bought, must be authorised by the person who bought such goods or services [30].

The definition of consumer under Section 2(1) (d) of the Consumer Protection Act does not cover persons who obtain service free of charge. On the question of services provided by the State free of charge, out of revenue collected in the form of taxes, the National Consumer Disputes Redressal Commission (NCDRC) held that taxes paid by public could not be held to be consideration within the meaning of Section 2(1) (d) of the

Consumer Protection Act [31].

The Commission observed, "In a welfare State, it is the responsibility of the government to provide adequate medical, health care and other facilities to all citizens... It is possible, indeed it is likely, that by opening up the definition of the term Consumer to all users of government hospitals, we may invite a flood of irresponsible litigation, especially since the National Commission as well as the State Commission and the District Forum are available free of cost to all complainants."

On the question of tax paid by citizens as consideration, within the meaning under the Section 2(1) (d) of the Consumer Protection Act, the Commission observed, "Tax is an imposition made for a public purpose without reference to any special benefit to be conferred on the payer of the tax. There is no element of quid pro quo between the tax payer and public authority levying the tax... . Again, a consideration is a valid consideration only if it is given freely. But, taxes are a compulsory levy being collected under the authority of law. They are an imposition and are not paid voluntarily or freely... . Again, generally speaking, consideration is an ingredient of an agreement or a contract ... In the case of State and citizen, there is no agreement or contract obliging the State to provide certain services and for the beneficiaries to pay for the same in the form of taxes."

Thus, consumer is (a) a patient who pays to get services of doctor/hospital; (b) any person who pays for the patient; (c) legal heirs/representatives of such patients; (d) spouse, parents and children of the patient.

Consumer Dispute: According to Section 2(1) (e), Consumer dispute means a dispute where the person against whom a complaint has been made, denies or disputes the allegations contained in the complaint.

Deficiency : According to Section 2(1) (g), Deficiency means any fault, imperfection, shortcoming or inadequacy in the quality, nature, and manner of performance which is required to be maintained by or under any law for the time being in force or has been undertaken to be performed by a person in pursuance of a contract or otherwise in relation to any service.

Service: According to Section 2(1) (o), Service means service of any description which is made available to potential users and includes the provision of facilities in connection with banking, financing, insurance, transport, processing, supply of electrical or other energy, boarding or lodging or both, (housing construction), [32] entertainment, amusement or the purveying of news or other information, but does not include the rendering of any service free of charge or under a contract of personal service.

Medical Profession Covered Under "Services"

The services rendered by medical professionals were not expressly or categorically included within the definition of services under the provisions of The Consumer Protection Act. But it is clear that two types of services i.e., service free of charge or the services under a personal contract were expressly excluded from the purview of the Act. Hence, the services, which are free of charge or under a contract of personal services, are not covered within the definition of the Services under the Act and any claim in respect of such services are out of the jurisdiction of the Fora.

It was held by the National Commission: "It is well established principle of statutory construction that where the words of the Statute are clear and unambiguous, they have to be given their full asset and their ambit cannot be cut down by reference to the preamble of the act, the statement of the objects and reasons appended to the Bill or to the debates and speeches on the floor of the Legislature/Parliament. The expression 'Service' has been defined in Section 2 (1)(o) of the Act as a meaning "service of any description" which is made available to the potential users. When Parliament has unambiguously defined the expression 'service' in such broad language giving it the widest amplitude, we see absolutely no warrant for cutting down and restricting the scope of definition to only services relating to "commercial transactions". Hence, we see no substance in the arguments advanced on behalf of the appellants and the interveners that services rendered by hospitals and members of Medical Profession for consideration will not constitute 'service' as defined in the Act because it does not relate to commercial transaction."

It is further held that in the case of hospitals, which provided treatment to patients for payment, we are unable to see how there is any element of personal service involved in such an arrangement. Hence, the activity of providing medical assistance for payment carried on by hospitals and members of the medical profession falls within he scope of the expression 'service' as defined in Section 2(1)(o) of the Act.

Finally, it has been decided by the Supreme Court of India in the landmark judgement that the medical profession is covered with the definition of services and are subject matter of the jurisdiction of the Consumer Forums [33].

The definition of service exempts two types of services, viz., (i) service rendered free of charge; and (ii) service rendered under a contract of personal service. However, in some situations these can be misused and exploited. Instances are not uncommon where the trader under the garb of rendering service free of charge forces his consumers to buy his products. Free camps for providing various treatments like eyes, ears etc., are generally being organised by pharmaceutical companies or with the help of these companies by private organisations. Outside these camps, the companies usually put their stalls, for selling their products. Generally the doctors treating the patients in these free camps advise the patients to buy medicines only of the sponsoring companies. This practice is nothing but an unfair trade practice, which usually escapes being noticed as unfair practised by the public and escapes from the penal provisions of the Act.

The second category of service which is exempted from the provisions of the Act, relates to a contract of personal service. The Act has not defined what is a contract of personal service.

The National Consumer Disputes Redressal Commission, while determining the question, whether the hiring of service of a tailor to whom a piece of cloth is entrusted by a customer for stitching against charges can be said to be under a contract of personal service under the Act, observed, [34] "Before we proceed further we may mention here that a distinction is to be drawn between contract for service and contract of service . In the one case the master can order or require what is to be done while in the other case he can not only order or require what is to be done but how itself it shall be done [35]."

The correct method of approach, therefore, in such cases would be to consider, whether having regard to the nature of the work there was due control and supervision by the employer or to use the words of Fletcher Moulton, L.J., at page 549 in *Simmons v. Health Laundry Co.* [36], "In my opinion it is impossible to lay down any rule of law distinguishing the one from the other. It is a question of fact to be decided by all circumstances of the case. The greater the amount of direct control exercised over the person rendering the services by the person contracting for them the stronger the grounds for holding it to be a contract of service, and similarly the greater the degree of independence of such control the greater the probability that the services rendered are of the nature of professional services and that the contract is one for service."

The National Commission after going through the facts and circumstances of the case held that the services rendered by the medical professionals do not come under a contract of personal service and observed:

"Of course in a narrow sense there is personal element in practically all services. However, it will be incorrect and even crude to call the professional or technical services as personal services."

What is Personal Service ?

The term "personal services" has not been defined under the Act but the same has been decided by Supreme Court and the

National Commission that 'Personal Service' stem from a master and servant relationship which is totally different from lawyer and client relationship or other professional or technical relationship. The reason for excluding rendering of service under a contract of personal service from the definition of service under the Act is obvious where such service can be turned out by the master at his will and therefore no occasion can arise for the master to complaint about the deficiency in rendering of service by the employee [37].

'Contract for Personal Service' distinguished from 'Contract of Personal Service'

A contract for services implies a contract whereby one party undertakes to render services e.g. professional or technical services, to or for another in the performance of which he is not subject to detailed direction and control but exercises professional or technical skill and uses his own knowledge and discretion. A 'contract of service' implies relationship of master and servant and involves an obligation to obey orders in the work to be performed and an obligation to obey orders in the work to be performed and as to its mode and manner of performance. We entertain no doubt that Parliamentary draftsman was aware of this well accepted distinction between "contract of service" and "contract for services" and has deliberately chosen the expression "contract of service" instead of the expression 'contract for services', in the exclusionary part of the definition of 'service' in Section 2(1)(o). The expression 'contract of personal service' in the exclusionary part of Section 2(1)(o) must, therefore, be construed as excluding the services rendered by an employee to his employer under the contract of personal service from the ambit of the expression 'service'. It is no doubt true that the rope between a medical practitioner and a patient carries within it certain degree of mutual confidence and trust and, therefore, the services rendered by the medical practitioners can be regarded as services of personal nature but since there is no relationship of master and servant between the doctor and the patient the contract between the medical practitioners and his patient cannot be treated as a contract of personal service but is a contract for services and the service rendered by the medical practitioners to his patient under such a contract is not covered by the exclusionary part of the definition of 'service' contained in Section 2(1)(o) of the Act [38].

What does Service "Free of Charge" Implies ?

The term "Service Free of Charge" has also not been defined under the Act but on the basis of the decision of the Supreme Court in Indian medical Association, supra, where the Apex Court observed that the medical practitioners, government hospitals/nursing homes and private hospitals/nursing homes broadly fall in three categories i.e., (1) where services are rendered free of charge to every body availing the said services, (2) where charges are required to be paid by every body availing the services, and (3) where charges are required to be paid by persons availing services but certain categories of persons who cannot afford to pay are rendered service of free of charge. The doctors and hospitals who render services without any charge whatsoever to every person, the person, who is availing such service would not fall within the ambit of 'service" under Section 2(1)(O) of the Act. The payment of a token amount for registration purposes only would not alter the position in respect of such doctors and hospitals. So far as the second category is concerned, since the services rendered on payment basis to all the persons they would clearly fall within the ambit of Section 2(1)(O) of the Act. The third category doctors and hospitals do provide free services to the patients belonging to the poor class but the bulk of service is rendered to the patient on payment basis. The expenses incurred for providing free service are met out of the income from the service rendered to the paying patients. The service rendered by such doctors and hospitals to paying patients undoubtedly fall within the ambit of Section 2(1)(O) of the Act. The service rendered to patients free of charge by the doctors and hospitals in category (3) is not excluded by virtue of exclusionary clause in Section 2(1)(O) of the Act.

What does not amount to Free Services ?

The complainant was operated upon, by the opposite party, in which a foreign body was left in the abdomen. He filed complaint alleging negligence. The opposite party contended that no fee was charged for operation but only received payment for medicines and operation theatre charges. It was held that the evidence of the opposite party itself would go to show that he had received a sum of Rs. 1,000/- from the parents of the complainant but he says that it was towards supply of medicines, operation theatre charges and room rent. These facts would go to show that the services rendered by the opposite party to the complainant were not completely free of charge as some services were for consideration. The commission followed the principles laid down in V.P. Shanta's case and held that it is clear that the services rendered by the doctors in the hospital falling under category where charges are required to be paid by persons availing services but certain categories of persons who cannot afford to pay are rendered service free of charges and therefore irrespective of the fact that the part of the service is free of charge, would nevertheless fall within the ambit of the expression 'service' as defined under Section 2(1)(O) of the Act. Having regard to the principles as laid down by the Hon'ble Supreme Court, the services rendered by the opposite party were for consideration and so the complainant is a 'consumer' under the provisions of the Act [39].

However, in the case where the complainants have nowhere stated in the complaint that they had paid any charges to respondent doctor of the hospital, the commissions, therefore, held that the services rendered by doctor were free of charge, if that is so, it will not be 'service' within the meaning of Section 2(1)(O) of the Act [40].

Government Servants under CGHS

Government servant under the Central Government Health Scheme is not a consumer within the meaning of Consumer

Protection Act, 1986 as defined in Section 2(1)(D) of the Act and the services rendered to him under the CGHS does not constitute service as defined under Section 2(1)(O) of the Act [41].

Government servant contributing for medical fund

The complainant was a Government Servant. While in service he was contributing monthly in medical fund which made him entitled to free medicine after retirement. He applied for re-imbursement of medical expenses, which were denied hence he filed the complainant. The opposite party raised a preliminary objection that complainant is not a consumer. It was held that a pensioner who avails of the facility of free supply of medicine by making monthly contribution while in service has hired the service in exchange for the contribution and is therefore a consumer, because the making of monthly contribution, while in service, is necessary for each Government servant to get the above benefit after retirement. Thus the opposite parties were rendering this service to all State Government Pensioners including the complainant for consideration. Consideration was received whilst the Government servant was in service and service to him was to be rendered after his retirement [42].

Thus, it is clear that so far as the special benefit and facility of supply of free medicines to a retired Government servant (pensioner) is concerned, the regular monthly contribution made by him, while in service, does constitute a consideration for the service to be rendered after his retirement, by way of supply of medicines free of charge which are needed by him in connection with his treatment whether as an outdoor patient or an indoor patient.

Tubectomy Operation: In another landmark judgement of the Supreme Court in the case of *State of Haryana and Ors. vs. Smt. Santra,* decided in April 2000, the Court held that in a country where the population is increasing by the tick of every second on the clock and the Government had taken up the family planning as an important programme for the implementation of which it had created mass awakening for the use of various devices including sterilisation operation, the doctor as also the State must be held responsible in damages if the sterilisation operation performed by him is a failure on account of his negligence which is directly responsible for another birth in the family, creating additional economic burden on the person who had chosen to be operated upon for sterilisation. Smt. Santra was a poor lady who already had seven children. She was already under considerable monetary burden. The unwanted child born to her has created additional burden for her on account of the negligence of the doctor who performed sterilisation operation upon her, and therefore she is clearly entitled to claim full damages from the State government to enable her to bring up the child till she attains puberty [43].

3.5.2 Enforcement Machinery under the Consumer Protection Act

The Consumer Protection Act is a welfare legislation which was enacted to provide for setting up of Consumer Protection Councils at the Central and the State levels [44] to promote and protect the rights of the consumer and a three-tier quasi judicial machinery for redressing consumer grievances [45].

Consumer Protection Councils : The Consumer Protection Act, 1986, envisages the establishment of the Central Consumer Protection Council [46] and the State Consumer Protection Councils [47] whose main objects are to promote and protect the rights of the consumers.

Central Consumers Protection Council: The Central Government is empowered to constitute the Central Consumer Protection Council, which shall consist of the following members [48]: (i) the Minister in-charge of Department of Food and Civil Supplies who shall be the Chairman of the Central Council; (ii) the Minister of State (where he is not holding independent charge) or Deputy Minister in the Department of Civil Supplies who shall be the Vice-chairman of the Central Council; (iii) the Ministers of Food and Civil Supplies or Ministers in-charge of Consumer Affairs in States; (iv) eight Members of Parliament-five from Lok Sabha and three from Rajya Sabha; (v) the Commissioner for Scheduled Castes and Scheduled Tribes; (vi) representatives of the Central Government Departments, autonomous organisations concerned with consumers interests- not exceeding twenty; (vii) representatives of the consumer organisations or consumers - not less than thirty five; (viii) representatives of women not less than ten; (ix) representatives of farmers, trade and industries - not exceeding twenty; (x) persons capable of representing consumer interests not specified above - not exceeding fifteen; (xi) the Secretary in the Department of Civil Supplies who shall be the member-secretary of the Central Council. The term of the Council is three years [49].

The Council may meet as and when necessary, but not less than three times a year [50].

Although the decisions of the Council are recommendatory in nature to the Central or State government, as the case may be, they may have a significant impact on the several authorities concerned with the matters of consumer protection [51]. The Central Consumer Protection Council in its meetings from time to time reviews the position of implementation of the Consumer Protection Act, 1986 and take the matter concerned with the appropriate Department or the Ministry concerned.

State Consumer Protection Councils : The State Governments are required to establish the Consumer Protection Councils for their respective States [52]. The State Council is to consist of such members as may be notified by the State Government by notification from time to time [53]. The objectives of every State Council [54] like the Central Council shall be to promote and protect within the State, the rights of the consumers. All the States have set up the Consumer Protection Councils under the Act. The State Councils have to take care of the implementation of the provisions of the Consumer Protection Act in their respective States. Their power in this regard is recommendatory in nature.

These Councils are expected to strengthen the consumer

movement in the country by providing forums at the Centre and the State where officials, consumer activists and policy makers can interact.

3.5.3 Machinery for Redressal of Consumer Disputes

The Act provides for the establishment of the three-tier quasi-judicial machinery for redressing consumer grievances.

District Forum

The Act envisages the establishment of a District Consumer Disputes Redressal Forum (DCDRC) also known as the District Forum in each District of the States and Union Territories. It is provided that each District Forum shall consists of president and two members, to be appointed by the State Government [55]. The President of the Forum is required to be a person who is, or has been qualified to be a District Judge. The other members of the Commission are to be the persons of ability, integrity and standing and having adequate knowledge and experience of, or have shown capacity in dealing with problems relating to economics, law, commerce, accountancy, industry, public affairs or administration. The District Commission is required to have two such members, one of whom shall be a woman (Section 10 and Section 16). The intention for having the members from fields other than the legal profession seems to be that the District Forum should be able to understand and appreciate the overall technical and social impact, while deciding the issues under the Act.

Tenure of Members of District Forum: Under the existing law, all the appointment of members are valid for a period of five years or upto the age of 65 years whichever is earlier, and shall not be eligible for reappointment [56]. The Act is silent regarding the tenure of the President but it may be implied that the provisions relating to members of the Forum apply to the President as well. However, a member may resign his office in writing under his hand addressed to the State Government and on such resignation being accepted, his office shall become vacant. The vacancy so caused may be filled by the appointment of a person possessing any of the qualifications mentioned above in relation to the category of member who had resigned.

Jurisdiction of the District Forum

The Jurisdiction may be defined to be the powers of the court to hear and determine a cause of adjudicate or exercise any Judicial Powers in relation to it. The question of jurisdiction is most relevant and important because any proceedings before the Fora if beyond the scope of Jurisdiction the same is not maintainable and even if any order or direction is passed the same becomes nullity. The place where original complaint can be filed depends upon two factors:

(a) The total pecuniary (monetary) value of the goods or services and the compensation claimed (if any).

(b) The geographical jurisdiction, i.e., where either the cause of action (reason for filing suit) arose or where the opposite party (defendant) actually and voluntarily resides or carries on business or personality works for gain.

The Jurisdiction of the District Forum has been defined in Section 11 of the Act. According to the contents of the said section and subject to other provisions of the Act, the District Forum shall have Jurisdiction to entertain complaints:

(1) Where the value of the goods or services and the compensation, if any, claimed does not exceed rupees five lacs.

(2) And within the local limits of whose Jurisdiction the opposite party or each of the opposite parties, where there are more than one, at the time of the institution of the complaint, actually and voluntarily resides or carries on business or has a branch office or personally works for gain; or any of the opposite parties, where there are more than one, at the time of the institution of the complaint, actually and voluntarily resides, or carries on business or has a branch office, or personally works for gain, provided that in such case either the permission of the District forum is given, or the opposite parties who do not reside, or carry on business or have a branch office, or personally work for gain, as the case may be acquiesce in such institution; or the

cause of action, wholly or in part, arises.

Procedure on receipt of complaint

The District Forum shall on receipt of a complaint-

(a) refer a copy of such complaint to the opposite party directing him to give his version of the case within a period of 30 days or such extended period not exceeding 15 days as may be granted by the district forums.

(b) where the opposite party on receipt of a copy of the complaint, denies or disputes the allegations contained in the complaint, or omits or fails to take any action to represent his case within the time given by the District Forum, the District Forum shall proceed to settle the consumer dispute, (i) on the basis of evidence brought to its notice by the complainant and the opposite party, where the opposite party denies or disputes the allegations contained in the complaint, (ii) on the basis of evidence brought to its notice by the complainant where the opposite party omits or fails to take any action to represent his case within the time given by the Forum, (iii) where the complainant or his authorised agent fails to appear before the District Forum on such day, the District Forum may in its discretion either dismiss the complaint in default or if a substantial portion of the evidence of the complainant has already been recorded, decide on its merits. Where the opposite party or its authorised agent fails to appear on the day of hearing the District Forum mat decide the complaint *ex-parte,* (iv) where any party to a complaint to whom time has been granted fails to produce his evidence or to cause the attendance of his witnesses, or to perform any other act necessary to the further progress of the complaint, for which time has been allowed, the District Forum may notwithstanding such default; 1. if the parties are present, proceed to decide the complaint forewith, or 2. if the parties or any of them is absent proceed as mentioned above, (v) the District Forum may, on such terms as it may think fit at any stage, adjourn the hearing of the complaint but not more than one adjournment shall ordinarily be given and the complaint should be decided within 90 days from the date of notice received by the opposite party where complaint does not require analysis or testing of the goods and within 150 days if it requires analysis or testing of the goods.

Findings of the District Forum

If, after the proceedings, the District Forum is satisfied that any of the allegations contained in the complaint about the services are proved, it shall issue an order to the opposite party directing him to do one or more of the following things:

(a) to return to the complainant the charges paid.

(b) pay such amount as may be awarded by it as compensation to the consumer for any loss or injury suffered by the consumer due to the negligence of the opposite party.

(c) to remove the deficiencies in the services in question.

(d) to provide for adequate costs to parties.

Appeal against the Orders of the District Forum : According to Section 15 of the Act, any person aggrieved by an order made by the District Forum can prefer an appeal against such order to the State Commission of the State, within a period of thirty days from the date of the order. However, the State Commission can entertain an appeal after the expiry of the said period of thirty days if it is satisfied that there was sufficient cause for the not filing it within that period.

State Commission

The second tribunal in the hierarchy of consumer grievance redressal agencies is the State Consumer Disputes Redressal Commission (SCDRC) at the State level also known as the State Commission. Each State is required to set up this commission with the prior approval of the Central Government [57].

Constitution of State Commission : The State Commission is to consist of a president and two other members, to be appointed by the State government. The president should be a person who is or has been a judge of a High Court, appointed by the State government [58]. The other two members should be persons of ability, integrity and standing and should have adequate knowledge or experience of, or have shown capacity in dealing with problems relating to economics, law, commerce, accountancy, industry, public affairs or administration, one of whom should be a women [59]. However, it is provided that the appointment of a sitting judge of a High Court to the Commission can be made only after consultation with the Chief Justice of that High Court [60]. The salary or honorarium and other allowances payable to the president and other members of the State Commission are to be prescribed by the State government [61]. The members of the State Commission retire at the age of 67 years or five years of service, whichever is early. The reappointment is expressly prohibited.

Jurisdiction of the State Commission

The Jurisdiction of the State Commission has been defined in Section 17 of the Act. According the contents of the said section, and Subject to the other provisions of this Act, the State Commission shall have Jurisdiction, (a) to entertain complaints where the value of the goods or services and compensation, if any, claimed exceeds rupees five lacs but does not exceed rupees twenty lacs; (b) to entertain appeals against the orders of any District Forum within the State; and (c) to entertain revision petitions against the District Forum and to call for the records and pass appropriate orders in any consumer dispute which is pending before or has been decided by any District Forum within the State, where it appears to the State Commission that such District Forum has exercised a jurisdiction not vested in it by law, or has failed to exercise a jurisdiction so vested or has acted in exercise of its jurisdiction illegally or with material irregularity.

Procedure to be followed by State Commission

Same as for District Forum

Appeal against the Orders of the State Commission : According to Section 19 of the Act, any person aggrieved by an order made by the State Commission on a complaint can prefer an appeal against such order to the National Commission within a period of thirty days from the date of the order. However, the

National Commission can entertain an appeal after the expiry of the said period of thirty days if it is satisfied that there was sufficient cause for not filling it within that period. The Central Government and the consumer organisations have been striving for expediting the constitution of the District Forums in each of the Districts and the State Commissions in each of the States. The Supreme Court has issued directions from time to time for speedy establishment of State Commission and District Forums in all the districts and the States [62].

As a result of the efforts done by the Central Government and the voluntary organisations and due to intervention of the Supreme Court, the constitution of the District Forums have been expedited. Table 3.1 gives the position of the constitution of various State Commissions and District Forums as on December 31, 2000.

Table 3.1: Position of Setting up Various State Commissions and District Forums as on December 31, 2000

Number of States and Union Territories in India	32
Number of State Commissions in India	32
Number of State Commissions not functioning	1
Number of Districts in India	553
Number of Districts Forums in India	555
Number of Districts Forums functioning	508
Number of Districts Forums not functioning	46

Source: Ministry of Civil Supplies, Consumer Affairs and Public Distribution, Government of India, New Delhi

National Commission

The Consumer Protection Act provides for the setting up of the National Consumer Disputes Redressal Commission (NCDRC) also known as the National Commission (NC) at the apex of the consumer disputes redressal agencies.

Composition: The National Commission is to consist of a President and four other members to be appointed by the Central

Government. The President should be a person who is, or has been, a judge of the Supreme Court. The members of the National Commission retire at the age of 70 years or after five years of service whichever is early. The reappointment is expressly prohibited.

Jurisdiction of the National Commission

The Jurisdiction of the National Commission has been defined in Section 21 of the Act. According to this section the National Commission, subject to the other provisions of this Act, shall have Jurisdiction to entertain complaints:

(a) Complaints where the value of the goods or services and compensation, if any, claimed exceeds rupees twenty lacs,

(b) Appeals against the order of any State Commission and;

(c) To entertain revision petition against the State Commission and, to call for the records and pass appropriate orders in any consumer dispute which is pending before or has been decided by any State Commission where it appears to the National Commission that such State Commission has exercised a jurisdiction so vested or has acted in exercise of the jurisdiction illegally or with material irregularity.

The above mentioned jurisdiction of the National Commission may be termed as original, appellate and revisional jurisdiction, respectively. The pecuniary jurisdiction is dependent upon the amount claimed and not on the basis of the value of the vehicle or goods [63].

Agreement Regarding Jurisdiction

Where there are two courts, which will have Jurisdiction, it is open to the parties to agree that only one of those courts will have Jurisdiction to try the suit [64]. The term of contract or agreement in respect of territorial Jurisdiction cannot invoke the Jurisdiction of the said court if no part of the cause of action can be said to have arisen within the territorial Jurisdiction of the said Court. The said term even if agreed between the parties, is not valid and enforceable [65].

The parties by an agreement cannot confer jurisdiction on a

Court, which has no Jurisdiction to try the case, but if more courts than one have got the Jurisdiction to try the case, the parties can mutually agree that the dispute between them shall be tried in one of such Courts [66].

The Act permits the restriction of the territorial Jurisdiction to one out of the two or more District Forums having concurrent Jurisdiction for the trial of consumer dispute by an express agreement of the parties [67].

Matter Already Decided by Civil Court

Consumer Forum cannot entertain the complaint where the matter has already decided by the Civil Court [68].

Resjudicata: A complaint was filed against the doctor but the doctor contended that no fees were taken. Hence the complaint was dismissed by the State Commission on the ground that the complainant is not a consumer. On appeal to the National Commission, the case was remanded back after finding that the complainant was consumer. The same objection was again raised before the State Commission. It was held if the opposite party was feeling dissatisfied with the order of the National Commission, it is open to him to challenge the same before the Supreme Court. But the same question cannot be re-agitated before the State Commission in view of the order of the National Commission that complainants are to be treated as consumer and the complaints are to be decided on merits [69].

It was observed that though the National Commission has, in some cases, come to the conclusion that if complicated questions arise, the parties should be relegated to their remedy before a Civil Court. But it will be for the Consumer Court concerned, as and when such cases relating to Doctors and hospitals come up, to decide for itself whether they should decide the case or to relegate the parties to their remedy before a Civil Court. It is not for High Court to entertain a Writ Petition and go into the question whether any case pending before the Consumer Court concerned involved complicated questions of fact or not, and decide whether the Consumer Court concerned should go ahead with the matter or not [70].

Procedure to be Followed by the National Commission

A complaint containing the following particulars shall be presented by the complainant in person or by his agent to the National Commission or be sent by registered post, addressed to the National Commission:

(a) The name, description and the address of the complainant;

(b) the name, description and address of the opposite party or parties, as the case may be, so far as they can be ascertained:

(c) the facts relating to the complaint and when and where it arose;

(d) documents in support of the allegations contained in the complaint;

(e) the relief which the complainant claims.

The remaining procedure and the procedure for hearing the appeal is similar to that for State Commission.

The District Forums, State Commissions and the National Commission formed under the Consumer Protection Act also have the powers of a Civil Court in respect of the following [71]:

(i) the summoning and enforcing attendance of any defendant or witnesses and examining the witness on oath;

(ii) the discovery and production of any document or other material object producible as evidence;

(iii) the reception of evidence on affidavits;

(iv) the requisitioning of the report of the concerned analysis or test from the appropriate laboratory or from any other relevant source;

(v) issuing of any commission for the examination of any witnesses; and

(vi) any other matter which may be prescribed.

The Central Government has further been given the power to confer more powers under the Civil Procedure Code on these consumer disputes redressal agencies in addition to those enumerated above. Every proceeding before the District Forum is deemed to be a judicial proceeding within the meaning of Sections 193 and 228 of the Indian Penal Code. No specific mention has been made of the powers of a State Commission, apart from the procedure to be followed by it. However, it may be safely assumed that the State Commission has the same powers under the Civil Procedure Code as have been expressly made applicable to the District Forum and the National Commission.

Under the rules framed by the Central Government, the National Commission, the State Commission and the District Forums have the additional power to require any person :

1. to allow examination of books of accounts, documents or commodities as may be required and to keep them under its custody for the purposes of the Act;

2. to furnish information which may be required for the purposes of the Act [72].

Enforcement of Orders and Penalties: The Act provides that every order of a District Forum, State Commission or the National Commission shall, if no appeal has been preferred against such order under the provisions of the Act, be final [73]. Every such order may be enforced by the District Forum, the State Commission or the National Commission, as the case may be, in the same manner as if it were a decree or order made by a court in a suit pending therein.

Where a trader or a person against whom a complaint is made fails or omits to comply with any order made by the District Forum, the State Commission or the National Commission as the case may be, such trader or person shall be punishable with imprisonment for a term which shall not be less than one month but which may extend to three years, or with fine which shall not be less than two thousand rupees but which may extend to ten thousand rupees, or with both. However, a term lesser than the minimum amount may be imposed, if the circumstances so require.

It is laudable that the Consumer Forums have been imposing

fine and imprisonment on persons for not complying with their directions. The District Forum, Faridabad, in its historic judgement imposed rupees ten thousand as damages on three respondent-officers of the telecommunications department, the General Manager, District Manager and S.D.O. to be deducted from their salaries in equal shares for committing perjury and making a false statement in the written statement [74]. The same District Forum, created a history of sorts, by imposing physical penalty of sentencing three officials of the telecommunication department to one month's simple imprisonment [75].

Provision of Appeals: All the orders passed by these Commissions are appelable, appeals can be filed against the decision of the District Forums to the respective State Commission and from the State Commissions to the National Commission. If any of the parties to the suit is still not satisfied, it can appeal to the Supreme Court (Section 23 of the CPA, 1986) against the decisions of the National Commission. All appeals are to be filed within 30 days of the date of order and each appeal is to be accompanied with a copy of the order.

The Supreme Court may entertain an appeal after 30 days if it is satisfied that there was sufficient cause for not filing it within that period.

Role of the Courts: Under the scheme of the Consumer Protection Act, 1986, the Supreme Court, the High Courts and the other Civil Courts have been assigned an important role. The Supreme Court has the power to decide appeals against certain decisions and orders passed by the National Consumer Dispute Redressal Commission [76].

The High Courts enjoy certain extraordinary powers conferred on them under the Constitution of India. Under Article 226 of the Constitution of India, every High Court has the power, within its territorial jurisdiction, to issue to any person or authority any direction, order, or appropriate writ for the enforcement of any fundamental rights or for any other purpose. The power of the High Courts is not in derogation of such power of the Supreme Court under Article 32 of the Constitution of India. Thus, the roles and powers of High Courts for the enforcement of provisions of the Consumer Protection Act, are mainly concerned with the issue of direction, order or an appropriate writ under Article 226 of the Constitution. In exercise of powers under Articles 226, High Courts have issued writs quashing proceedings before the District Forums when they exceeded their jurisdiction [77].

In *P.P. Ismail v. Kerala State Consumer Disputes Redressal Commission and Ors.*, [78], the Kerala High Court observed: "though the National Commission has, in some cases, come to the conclusion that if complicated questions arise, the parties should be relegated to their remedy before a Civil Courts. But it will be for the Consumer Court concerned, as and when such cases relating to Doctors and hospitals come up, to decide for itself whether they should decide the case or to relegate the parties to their remedy before a Civil Courts. It is nor for High Court to entertain a writ petition and go into the question whether any case pending before the Consumer Court concerned involves complicated questions of fact or not, and decide whether the Consumer Court concerned should go ahead with the matter or not."

Under the scheme of the Consumer Protection Act, 1986, the role of Civil Courts (Courts below High Courts) is limited only to execute the orders passed by the District Forums or the State Commissions or the National Commission, in case the latter is unable to execute the same. As provided in the Act, every order made by the District Forum, the State Commission or the National Commission, can be enforced by the District Forums, the State Commission or the National Commission, as the case may be, in the same manner as if it were a decree or order made by a court in a suit pending therein and it shall be lawful for the District Forum, the State Commission, or the National Commission to send, in the event of its inability to execute it, such order to the Court within the local limits of jurisdiction as given below: (i) in the case of an order against a company, where the registered office of the company is situated, or (ii) in the case of an order against any other person, the place where the person concerned voluntarily resides or carries on business or personally works for gain, is situated.

The Court to which the order is so sent shall execute the order as if it were a decree or order sent to it for execution [79].

3.5.4 Limitation Period: Ordinarily complaints are to be filed within two years form the date on which cause of action arose (Section 24A). According to Section 24(A)(i) and (ii), the respective Commission may condone the delay (after recording the reasons), if the complainant satisfies them that he had sufficient reasons for not filing the complaints within such period. No such complaint shall be entertained unless the National Commission, the State Commission or the District Forum, as the case may be, records its reasons for condoning such delay.

In *Mukund Lal Ganguly vs. Dr. Abhijit Ghosh and Ors.* III (1995)CPJ 64, the complainant got his eye operated in 1989 but the complaint was filed on 11.01.1994. The opposite party raised a preliminary objection that the complaint has been filed after more than two years from the date of his blindness and as such the case is barred by limitation. It was held that although he got his certificate of blindness as a handicapped person on 18.12.1989, he was still in the faint hope of recovering his vision by a further operation and it was only after the operation that he finally came to know that he had permanently lost his sight. The cause of action for filing the complaint arose after that date. The complaint was discharged on 21.1.1992 and if limitation is counted from that date, the complaint is within the period of limitation. Further, even if the period of limitation is counted from before that date, we think that there are reasonable grounds to entertain this complaint by condoning the delay as in our opinion the complainant had sufficient cause for not filing the complaint within the period of limitation.

3.5.5 Time Limit of Disposal: Although nothing has been specified in the Act per se but the rules and regulations made under the powers conferred to the Central Government and State Government [under Section 30 (1) and (2)] indicate that complaints shall as far as possible be decided within a period of three months from the date of notice received by the opposite party where the complaint does not require analysis or testing of commodity, and within five months where such analysis or testing is required.

The National Commission and the State Commissions are required to decide the appeal as far as possible within 90 days from the first date of hearing. The main thrust of the Act is to provide simple, speedy and inexpensive redressal to an aggrieved consumer. Thus, to ensure speedy disposal of consumer grievances, the above provisions have been incorporated in the Act.

3.5.6 Reliefs for Deficiency in Service

The reliefs that could be granted for deficiency in service are (i) return of charges paid by the complainant, (ii) payment of such amount as may be awarded as compensation to the consumer for any loss or injury suffered by the consumer due to negligence of the opposite party; (iii) removal of defect or deficiency in the service in question; and (iv) to provide for adequate costs to parties

3.5.7 Action against Frivolous or Vexatious Complaints: To discourage frivolous or vexatious litigation, the Act has provided the provision for dismissal of such complaints with costs not exceeding ten thousand rupees under Section 26.

Section 26 : "Where a complaint instituted the District Forum, the State Commission or the National Commission, as the case may be, is found to be frivolous or vexatious, it shall, for reasons to be recorded in writing, dismiss the complaint and make an order that the complainant shall pay to the opposite party such cost, not exceeding ten thousand rupees, as may be specified in the order."

The complaints without evidence or material are also considered as frivolous or vexatious. In *Sudhakar Dattatraya vs. The Nirma Chemical Works* [80] it was observed, "The complainant had filed the complaint without any evidence or material except his say. It is almost of the nature of being frivolous and therefore not maintainable."

It was observed by the National Commission that by filing a complaint seeking to recover the compensation of Rs. 55,99,000 from the opposite party the motive of the complainant was only to indulge in speculative litigation taking undue advantage of the fact that no court fee is payable for institution of a case under the C.P. Act. It was also noted that such false and vexatious complaint being lodged before the Consumer Forum with a view to harass and black mail those who supply the goods and provide services to the community should be discouraged. The complaint was dismissed with cost of Rs. 10,000/- under Section 26 of C.P. Act [81].

The National Commission observed that the complaint was frivolous and was a misuse of the Consumer Protection Act causing harassment and expense to the respondent hospital in defending itself against the complaint and the complaint is malafide, vexatious and frivolous and that the hospital which is run by a public trust, had to incur heavy expenditure for contesting the complaint. In such circumstances, the National Commission dismissed the complaint with the direction that the complainant shall pay a sum of Rs. 10,000/- as costs to the respondent hospital [82].

3.5.8 Penalties: Under Section 27, when a trader or a person against whom a complaint is made (or complainant) fails or omits to comply with any order made by the District Forum, the State Commission or the National Commission, as the case may be, such trader or person (or complainant) shall be punishable with imprisonment for a term which shall not be less than one month but which may extend to three years, or with fine which shall not be less than two thousand rupees but which may extend to ten thousand rupees, or with both.

It is provided that the District Forum, the State Commission or the National Commission, as the case may be, may, if it is satisfied that the circumstances of any case so require, impose a sentence of imprisonment or fine, or both, for a term lesser than the minimum term and the amount lesser than the minimum amount, specified in this Section.

3.5.9 The Supreme Court Judgement in *Indian Medical Association v. V.P. Shantha* [83]. The landmark judgement by the Supreme Court on November 13, 1995, stating that the medical services to patients for which fees are charged, come under the purview of the Consumer Protection Act, 1986, has put a curtain on the long-drawn-out debate between doctors and consumers on the issue. The judgement given by Justice Kuldip Singh, Justice S. C. Agrawal and Justice B.L. Hansaria, made doctors accountable for any act of medical negligence and ruled that they could be sued for compensation under the Consumer Protection Act, 1986. Some pertinent observations made by the Supreme Court in the above-mentioned case are reproduced hereby:

(1) The Supreme Court observed that in the matter of professional liability, profession differ from other occupation for the reason that the professional operates in a sphere where success cannot be achieved in every case and very often success or failure depends upon factors beyond the professional mans control. In devising a rational approach to professional liabilities which must provide proper protection to the consumers while allowing for the factors mentioned above, the approach of the Court is to require that professional men should possess a certain minimum degree of competence and that they should exercise reasonable care in the discharge of their duties. Medical practitioners do not enjoy any immunity and they can be sued in the Law of Contract or the Law of Torts on the grounds that they had failed to exercise reasonable skill and care. The Court further, held that while immunity from damages was enjoyed by

certain professions on the grounds of public interest, the trend today was narrowing such immunity.

(2) The judges observed that the legal system has to do justice to both patients and doctors. The fears of medical profession should be taken into account while the legitimate claims of the patients cannot be ignored. It would be a mistake to think of doctors and hospitals as easy targets for the dissatisfied patients. It is still very difficult to raise an action of medical negligence. A patient who has been injured by the act of medical negligence deserves compensation for the loss of future earning and the cost of medical treatment. After all, there is no difference in legal theory between a person injured through medical negligence and industrial or motor accident.

(3) The Supreme Court did not agree with the contention that the composition of the District Forum, the State Commission and the National Commission is such that they cannot fully appreciate the complex issues. According to the apex Court, in the matter of constitution of the District Forum, the State Commission and the National Commission, the CPA, 1986, combines with legal competence, the merits of lay decision-making by members having, knowledge and experience in dealing with problems relating to various fields which are connected with the object and purpose of the CPA, 1986, namely, protection of the interests of the Consumers. Moreover, there is further safeguard of an appeal against the order made by the District Forum to the State Commission and against the order made by the State Commission to the National Commission and further, appeal to the Supreme Court against the order of the National Commission. According to the Supreme Court, it could not, therefore, be said that the composition of the Consumer Disputes Redressal Agencies is such as to render them unsuitable for adjudication on issues arising in a complaint regarding deficiency in service rendered by a medical practitioner.

(4) Regarding the contention that the proceedings involving negligence in the matter of rendering services by a medical

practitioner would raise complicated questions requiring evidence of experts to be recorded and that the procedure which is followed under the CPA for determination of consumer disputes is summary in nature and not suitable for determination of complicated questions, the Supreme Court held that there was no doubt that sometimes complicated questions requiring the recording for evidence of experts may arise in a complaint about deficiency in service based on the ground of negligence in rendering medical services by a medical practitioner; but this would not be so in all complaints about deficiency in rendering services by a medical practitioner. There may be cases which do not raise such complicated questions and the deficiency in service may be due to obvious faults which can be easily established such as removal of the wrong limb or the performance of an operation on the wrong patient or giving injection or drug to which the patient is allergic without looking into the out-patient card containing the warning or use of wrong gas during the course of an anaesthesia or leaving inside the patient's body, other items of operating equipment after surgery.

According to the Supreme Court, the issues arising in the complaints in such cases could be speedily disposed of by the procedure that was being followed by the Consumer Disputes Redressal Agencies and there was no reason why complaints regarding deficiency in service in such cases should not be adjudicated by the Agencies established under the Act. According to the Court, in complaints involving complicated issues requiring recording of evidence of experts, the complainants could be asked to approach the Civil Court for appropriate relief. Section 3 of the Consumer Protection Act, 1986 which prescribes that the provisions of this Act shall be in addition to and not in derogation of the provisions of any other law for the time being in force, preserves the right of the consumer to approach the Civil Courts for necessary relief.

The operative part of the judgement in given below :

1. Service rendered to a patient by a medical practitioner

(except where the doctor renders service free of charge to every patient or under a contract of personal service), by way of consultation, diagnosis and treatment, both medicinal and surgical, would fall within the ambit of service as defined in Section 2(1) (o) of the Act.

2. The fact that the medical practitioners belong to the medical profession and are subject to the disciplinary control of the Medical Council of India and/or State Medical Councils, constituted under the Indian Medical Council Act, would not exclude the service rendered by them from the ambit of the Act.

3. A contract of personal services has to be distinguished from a contract for personal service . In the absence of a relationship of master and servant between the patient and medical practitioner, the service rendered by a medical practitioner to the patient cannot be regarded as service rendered under a contract of personal service . Such service is service rendered under a contract for personal service and is not covered by exclusionary clause of the definition of service contained in Section 2(1)(o) of the Act.

4. The expression contract of personal service in Section 2(1) (o) of the Act cannot be confined to contracts for employment of domestic servants only and the said expression would include the employment of a medical officer for the purpose of rendering medical service to the employer. The service rendered by a medical officer to his employer under the contract of employment would be outside the purview of service as defined in Section 2(1) (o) of the Act.

5. Service rendered free of charge by a medical practitioner attached to a hospital/nursing home or a medical officer employed in a hospital/nursing home where such services are rendered free of charge to everybody, would not be service as defined in Section 2(1) (o) of the Act. The payment of a token amount for registration purpose only at the hospital/nursing home would not alter the position.

6. Service rendered at a non-government hospital/nursing home where no charge whatsoever is made from any person availing the service and all patients (rich and poor) are given free service, is outside the purview of the expression service as defined in Section 2(1) (o) of the Act. The payment of a token amount for registration purpose only at the hospital/nursing home would not alter the position.

7. Service rendered at a non-government hospital/nursing home where charges are required to be paid by the persons availing such services falls within the purview of the expression service as defined in Section 2(1) (o) of the Act.

8. Service rendered at a non-government hospital/nursing home where charges are required to be paid by persons who are in a position to pay and persons who cannot afford to pay are rendered service free of charge would fall within the ambit of the expression service as defined in Section 2(1) (o) of the Act irrespective of the fact that the service is rendered free of charge to persons who are not in a position to pay for such services. Free service, would also be service and the recipient a consumer under the Act.

9. Service rendered at a government hospital / health centre / dispensary where no charge whatsoever is made from any person availing the services and all patients (rich and poor) are given free service, is outside the purview of the expression service as defined in Section 2(1) (o) of the Act. The payment of a token amount for registration purpose only at the hospital/nursing home would not alter the position.

10. Service rendered at a government hospital / health centre / dispensary where services are rendered on payment of charges and also rendered free of charge to other persons availing such services would fall within the ambit of the expression service as defined in Section 2(1) (o) of the Act irrespective of the fact that the service is rendered free of free of charge to persons who do not pay for such service. Free service would also be service and the recipient a consumer under the Act.

11. Service rendered by a medical practitioner or

hospital/nursing home cannot be regarded as service rendered free of charge, if the person availing the service has taken an insurance policy for medical care where under the charges for consultation, diagnosis and medical treatment are borne by the insurance company and such service would fall within the ambit of service as defined in Section 2(1) (o) of the Act.

12. Similarly, where, as a part of the conditions of service, the employer bears the expenses of medical treatment of an employee and his family members dependent on him, the service rendered to such an employee and his family members by a medical practitioner or a hospital/nursing home would not be free of charge and would constitute service under Section 2(1) (o) of the Act.

Thus, the medical practitioners, Government hospitals/nursing homes and private hospitals/nursing homes (hereinafter called doctors and hospitals) are broadly fall in three categories:

(a) where services are rendered free of charge to everybody availing the said services. (b) where charges are required to be paid by persons availing the services, and (c) where charges are required to be paid by persons availing services but certain categories of persons who cannot afford to pay are rendered service free of charges.

Doctors and hospitals who render services without any charge whatsoever to every person availing the service would not fall within the ambit of service under Section 2(1) (o) of the Act. The payment of a token amount for registration purposes only, would not alter the position in respect of such doctors and hospitals. So far as the second category is concerned, since the service is rendered on payment basis to all the persons they would clearly fall within the ambit of Section 2(1) (o) of the Act. The third category of doctors and hospitals do provide free service to some of the patients belonging to the poor class but the bulk of the service is rendered to the patients on payment basis. The expenses incurred for providing free service are met out of the income from the service rendered to the paying patients. The service rendered by such doctors and hospitals to paying patients undoubtedly fall within the ambit of Section 2(1) (o) of the Act.

Adverting to the individual doctors employed and serving in the hospital, the Supreme Court was of the view that such doctors working in the hospital nursing homes/dispensaries whether government or private, belonging to categories (ii) and (iii) above would be covered by the definition of service under the CPA, 1986 and as such were amendable to the provisions of the Act along with the management of the hospital etc. and severally.

3.5.10 Functioning of the Consumer Courts

The summary of cases disposed of by the National Consumer Disputes Redressal Commission is presented in Table 3.2. It can be observed from the Table that a large number of complaints of all types including those relating to deficiency of medical services, were filed (22,275) before the National Commission since its inception till March 31, 2001.

In all, 12659 complaints were disposed of. The disposed rate being 56.8 per cent and 9616 complaints (43.2 per cent) still pending with the Commission as on March 31, 2001.

The year-wise position of institution of complaints against deficiency in medical services by the National commission is shown in Table 3.3.

Further, Table 3.3 shows that there is substantial increase in the number of complaints received and appeals filed relating to deficiency in medical services after the landmark judgement of the Supreme Court in the above mentioned case. The table shows that in all 308 cases i.e., 9.95 per cent were filed against deficiency in medical services as original petition (OP) and 230 cases (4.05 per cent) as first appeals (FA).

The position of complaints filed before the Delhi State Consumer Disputes Redressal Commission is shown in Table 3.4. As shown in the Table, 4373 original complaints were instituted before the Delhi State Commission, since its inception till December 31, 2000, out of which 2845 (65.0 percent) were disposed of during the period. Moreover, 7336 (68.24 percent) of

Table 3.2: Summary of Cases Disposed of by the National Consumer Disputes Redressal Commission (From Inception till March 31, 2001)

Nature of the cases	1986 to 1994	1995	1996	1997	1998	1999	2000	2001	Total
Original Complaints (A)									
Filed during the year	1164	208	300	304	300	375	443	106	3200
Disposed off so far	1114	77	56	51	72	80	147	23	1620
Pending	50	131	244	253	228	295	296	83	1580
First Appeal (B)									
Filed during the year	2596	629	695	565	387	486	322	89	5769
Disposed off so far	2364	167	117	95	84	63	108	19	3017
Pending	232	462	578	470	303	423	214	70	2752
Revision Petition (C)									
Files during the year	2536	1123	1437	1500	1344	2360	2282	724	13306
Disposed off so far	2536	1123	1207	1127	718	751	364	196	8022
Pending	--	--	230	373	626	1609	1918	528	5284
Total Complaints Filed (A+B+C)									**22275**
Total Complaints Disposed of so far (A+B+C)									**12659**
Pending (A+B+C)									**9616**

Source : Compiled from the office of the National Consumer Disputes Redressal Commission, New Delhi.

the appeal cases were also disposed of till December 31, 2000.

A summary of the original complaints received against deficiency in medical services by the Delhi State Commission since its inception till December 31, 2000, is presented in Table 3.5. It can be observed from Table 3.5 that the number of complaints against deficiency in medical services instituted in Delhi State Commission has increased after the landmark

Table 3.3: Complaints pertaining to Deficiency in Medical Services before the National Consumer Disputes Redressal Commission (Since inception till December 31, 2000)

S. No.	Year	Original Petition			First Appeal		
		Total	Medical	Percent	Total	Medical	Percent
1.	1988	8	--	--	6	--	--
2.	1989	45	1	2.22	25	1	4.0
3.	1990	49	1	2.04	109	--	--
4.	1991	121	4	3.31	296	8	2.70
5.	1992	291	21	5.12	625	13	2.08
6.	1993	350	39	11.14	730	21	2.73
7.	1994	300	13	4.33	805	15	1.86
8.	1995	208	8	3.85	629	16	2.54
9.	1996	300	31	10.33	695	3	4.75
10.	1997	304	57	18.75	565	38	6.73
11.	1998	300	50	16.66	387	27	6.98
12.	1999	375	56	14.93	486	26	6.30
13.	2000	443	37	8.35	322	32	10.00
Total		**3094**	**308**	**9.95**	**5680**	**230**	**4.05**

Source : Compiled from the office of the National Consumer Disputes Redressal Commission, New Delhi.

Table 3.4: Summary of Cases Handled by the Delhi State Consumer Disputes Redressal Commission (since inception till December 31, 2000)

Nature of Cases	Complaints	
	Number	Percent
Total No. of original complaints Instituted (A)		
Received	4373	
Disposed of	2845	65.06
Pending	1528	34.94
Total No. of Appeals Revision Instituted (B)		
Received	10,750	
Disposed of	7,336	68.24
Pending	3,414	31.76
Total No. of Complaints (A+B)	15,123	
Total Disposed of (A+B)	10,181	67.32
Pending	4,942	32.68

Source: Compiled from the Office of the Delhi State Commission, New Delhi.

Table 3.5: Complainant Regarding Deficiency in Medical Services Filed Before the Delhi State Consumer Disputes Redressal Commission (since inception till December 2000)

S. No.	Year	Complaints (original jurisdiction)		
		Total	Medical	Percent
1.	1988	13	--	--
2	1989	26	--	--
3.	1990	139	3	2.15
4.	1991	352	6	1.70
5.	1992	651	29	4.45
6.	1993	685	35	5.10
7.	1994	364	15	4.12
8.	1995	281	12	4.27
9.	1996	334	32	9.58
10.	1997	382	31	8.12
11.	1998	386	33	8.55
12.	1999	402	32	7.96
13.	2000	346	41	11.84

Source: Compiled from the office of the Delhi State Consumer Disputes Redressal Commission, New Delhi.

judgement of the Supreme Court in the *Indian Medical Association v. V.P. Shantha* in 1995. Out of the total complaints received, 9.58 percent were against deficiency in medical services in the year 1996, alone. The corresponding figures for the year 1999 and 2000 are 7.96 percent and 11.84 percent, respectively.

The comparative position of the number of complaints received and their disposal by the Consumer Disputes Redressal Forums at all the three levels (i.e. National, State and District) is shown in the Table 3.6.

It can be observed from the Table that approximately 57 percent of the complaints are disposed of up to March 31, 2001 and 43 percent are still pending.

The disposal rate of the Delhi State Commission is 63.83 percent and that of District Forums of Delhi is 81.27 percent.

Table 3.6: Complaints Handled by the Consumer Courts : National Commission, State Commissions and District Forums

Nature of Cases	Complaints	
	Number	Percent
National Commission (Since inception till March 31, 2001)		
Cases filed	22,275	
Cases disposed of	12,659	56.83
Cases Pending	9,616	43.17
Delhi State Commission (Since inception till March 31, 2001)		
Cases filed	12,205	
Cases disposed of	7,791	63.83
Cases pending	4,414	36.17
District Forums, Delhi (Since inception till December 31, 2000)		
Cases filed	101,356	
Cases disposed of	82,367	81.27
Cases pending	18,989	18.73
Percentage of cases disposed of within 90 days as on 30.6.2000		7.63

Source: Collected from the office of the National Consumer Disputes Redressal Commission, New Delhi.

Table 3.7 gives a detailed account of the cases filed, disposed of and pending in the National Commission and various State Commissions. Table 3.8 depicts various cases filed/disposed of and pending in various district courts.

3.5.11 Approach of the Consumer Courts: In order to evaluate the approach of the Consumer Courts in deciding cases relating to deficiency in medical services, cases decided by the National Commission and cases decided by various State Commissions (since their inception till January 31, 2001) have been reviewed in the present study.

Table 3.7: Statement of Cases Filed/Disposed of/Pending in the National Commission and State Commissions

Name of State	Cases filed since inception	Cases disposed of since inception	Cases disposed of within 90 days	% of disposal within 90 days	Cases disposed of within 150 days	% of disposal within 150 days	Period of reporting
National Commission	22276						31.3.2001
Andhra Pradesh	12287	10075	2416	23.98	1726	17.13	31.3.2001
Arunachal pradesh	19	13	0	0.00	2	15.38	31.3.2000
Assam	1332	656	93	14.18	68	10.37	30.9.2000
Bihar	6712	2596	No information				30.6.2000
Goa	1244	1052	248	23.57	107	10.17	31.3.2001
Gujarat	8067	4672	No information				30.9.2000
Haryana	12268	9088	3285	36.15	2235	24.59	31.3.2001
Himachal Pradesh	4876	3480	893	25.66	349	10.03	31.3.2001
Jammu & Kashmir	3232	3232	No information				31.3.1999
Karnataka	10008	7425	812	10.94	472	6.36	31.3.2001
Kerala	14477	12365	4903	39.65	3981	32.20	30.9.2000
Madhya Pradesh	11046	10603	No information				30.9.2000
Maharashtra	17979	9947	770	7.74	2190	22.20	31.12.99
Manipur	62	62	No information				31.5.2000
Meghalaya	84	60	9	15.00	10	16.67	30.9.2000

Contd....

Mizoram	51	24	15	62.50	2	8.33	31.12.2K
Nagaland	40	15	10	66.67	0	0.00	31.3.2000
Orissa	8513	4255	181	4.25	151	3.55	31.3.2001
Punjab	8392	6225	1158	18.60	1228	19.73	31.3.2001
Rajasthan	20063	7752	404	5.21	806	10.40	31.3.2001
Sikkim	18	16	No information				30.9.2000
Tamil Nadu	12522	9551	2774	29.04	2915	30.52	31.3.2001
Tripura	494	196	89	45.41	35	17.86	31.3.2001
Uttar Pradesh	29982	6785	237	3.49	440	6.48	31.3.2001
West Bengal	6677	4291	55	21.49	19	0.44	31.12.2K
A&N Islands	26	28	No information				31.3.2000
Chandigarh	2656	2232	81	3.63	39	1.75	30.9.2000
D&N Haveli	0	0	0	0	0	0	
Daman & Diu	5	2	No information				31.12.2K
Delhi	12205	7791	No information				31.3.2000
Lakshadweep	9	9	0	0	1	11.11	31.3.2001
Pondicherry	577	546	199	36.45	182	33.33	31.3.2001
Total	**228198**	**118969**	**18632**	**15.66**	**16958**	**14.25**	

Table 3.8: Statement of Cases Filed/Disposed of/Pending in Districts

Name of State	Cases filed since inception	Cases disposed of since inception	Cases Pending	% of disposal	As on
Andhra Pradesh	123377	107938	15439	87.49	31.3.2001
Arunachal pradesh	189	160	29	84.66	31.3.2000
Assam	7285	6260	1025	85.93	30.9.2000
Bihar	51593	35373	16220	68.56	30.9.2000
Goa	3869	3195	674	82.58	30.4.2001
Gujarat	65212	45960	19252	70.48	30.9.2000
Haryana	88963	68594	20369	77.10	31.3.2001
Himachal Pradesh	23369	18569	4800	79.46	31.3.2001
Jammu & Kashmir	10436	8247	2189	79.02	31.3.1999
Karnataka	61671	55801	5870	90.48	31.3.2001
Kerala	113722	107582	6140	94.60	31.3.2001
Madhya Pradesh	69711	62566	7145	89.75	31.12.2000
Maharashtra	98407	77892	20515	79.15	31.12.1999
Manipur	803	774	29	96.39	31.5.2000
Meghalaya	242	199	43	82.23	30.6.1999
Mizoram	1087	911	176	83.81	31.12.2000
Nagaland	60	21	39	35.00	31.3.2000
Orissa	37893	32073	5820	84.64	30.9.2000

Contd...

Punjab	48119	42810	5309	88.97	31.3.2001
Rajasthan	153117	137398	15719	89.73	31.3.2001
Sikkim	113	105	8	92.92	31.3.2001
Tamil Nadu	58686	51899	6787	88.44	31.3.2001
Tripura	882	785	97	89.00	30.9.2000
Uttar Pradesh	242776	176897	65879	72.86	31.3.2000
West Bengal	35639	32040	3599	89.90	31.3.2000
A&N Islands	217	194	23	89.40	31.3.2000
Chandigarh	18701	15401	3300	82.35	31.3.2001
D&N Haveli	33	23	10	69.70	31.12.1999
Daman & Diu	62	37	25	59.68	30.9.2000
Delhi	88843	66908	21935	75.31	31.3.2000
Lakshadweep	35	35	0	100.00	31.3.2001
Pondicherry	1782	1746	36	97.98	31.3.2001
Total	**1406894**	**1158393**	**248501**	**82.34**	

Approach of the National Commission: A summary of the major cases decided by the National Commission against deficiency in medical services, since inception till January 31, 2001, is given in Table 3.9.

A summary account of the review of the cases pertaining to deficiency in medical services by the National Commission is given below:

It is observed that out of 53 cases, 13 cases, (24.53 per cent) was decided in favour of the patients. However, in 32 cases (60.38 per cent) the National Commission held that there was no deficiency in providing medical services by the doctor or the health institution. Five cases were remanded back to the State Commissions for fresh consideration and for giving opportunity to both the parties to produce further evidence and three cases were related to free health service provided by the government hospitals which were not covered under the CPA, 1986.

Moreover, death was not found to be the main ground for filing complaints against doctors in 60.38 per cent of cases (32 out of 53 cases). Furthermore, complaints were largely related to deficiency in treatment in surgical operation (62.26 per cent i.e. 33 out of 53 cases) as against non-surgical treatment (20 out of 53 cases).

Cases relating to safeguards against misuse of consumer protection measures: The cases reviewed indicate quite clearly that the fear in the mind of some of the doctors that the law is against them is unjustified. Also frivolous or vexatious complaints for blackmailing or humiliating any doctor have been dealt seriously and strong action were taken against such complainants by the Consumer Courts

The National Commission has also awarded costs to the complainants on the ground of unfounded allegations raised by the complainants in the case of *A. Narain Rao vs. Dr. G. Ramakrishna Reddy and Anr.* and *Miss Gurpreet Kaur vs. Dr. R. K. Butani*. In the first case, the Court ordered a cost of Rs. 5000/- and in the second case, a cost of Rs. 7500/-.

Table 3.9

Summary of Major Cases relating to Deficiency in Medical Services Decided by the National Commission
(Since inception up to December 31, 2000)

Sr. No.	Case No./Year and source	Case Title	Basis of Complaint	Final order	
				Date	Summary
1.	F.A.No.2/1989 I (1992) CPJ 259 (NC)	Consumer Unity and Trust Society, Jaipur v. The State of Rajasthan & Ors.	Negligence in operation; complainant underwent tubectomy operation at govt. hospital, complications developed; became physically invalid. State Commission, Jaipur held, free services not covered under the CPA. Hence, appeal made against the order.	15.12.89	Held, persons who avail of the facilities of medical treatment in govt. hospitals are not consumers and the said service can not be regarded as service 'hired' for 'consideration'; appeal rejected.
2.	F.A.No.3/1990	M.A. Azeez v. Naguru Jajana	Negligence in medical services. Boy died; State Commission allowed the complaint. Appeal made against the order.	5.4.90	Held, legal representatives entitled to claim compensation for death on account of negligence of doctors; appeal dismissed.
3.	O.P. No.15 and 16/1989 I (1992) CPJ 113 (NC)	Marble Roosevelt v. State of Kerala	Deficiency and negligence in treatment. Patient suffered heart attack and became semi-conscious for 1½ years and had been reduced to a state of vegetable.	10.7.90	Held, free services not covered under the Act; complaint dismissed.
4.	F.A.No.96/1990 II (1991) CPJ 202 (NC)	S.K. Abdul Sukur v. State of Orissa & Ors.	Deficiency in transfusion of blood and negligence in blood group test; patient died. State Commission held, competent Forum in this case is Civil Court as oral evidence and cross-examination is necessary. Appeal made against the order.	5.4.91	Held, State Commission was in error in denying to adjudicate upon the merits of the complaint; remanded the case to it for fresh disposal in accordance with law.

5.	O.P.No.11/1991 II (1992) CPJ 372 (NC)	Vinitha Ashok v. Lakshmi Hospital and Ors.	Negligence in removal of uterus at young age.	8.5.91	Held, doctor acted with due care and competence and in order to save life; uterus was removed; complaint dismissed with costs.
6.	(1991) I CPC 78	Mappoyan v. Premavathy Illango	Deficiency in providing medical services.	1991	Held, medical service for a 'consideration' is a service within the ambit of the Act. and complainant is a consumer under Section 2(1)(d) of Act; complaint allowed.
7.	F.A.No.114/1991	Sunil Blood Bank and Transfusion Centre v. Shri Naresh Kumar & Anr.	Deficiency in medical services. Transfusion of contaminated blood by virus Hepatitis B. State Commission, Delhi, allowed compensation of Rs.20,000. Order was passed by State Commission ex-parte. Appeal made against the order.	10.1.92	Case remanded to State Commission to disposed of afresh after giving adequate opportunities to both parties to adduce oral and documentary evidence.
8.	O.P.No.84/1991 II (1992) CPJ 391 (NC)	Renu Jain & Ors. v. Escorts Heart Institute & Research Centre	Deficiency in service on the part of hospital in treating and taking post-operative care; complainant's husband undergone coronary bypass surgery; got infection in leg; died.	10.4.92	No negligence proved in diagnosis and treatment in hospital; the cause of death was brainstem haemorrhage, not infection in leg; complaint dismissed.
9.	F.A.48/1991 I (1992) CPJ 302 (NC)	Cosmopolitian Hospital v. Smt. Vasantha P. Nair & Ors.	Deficiency and negligence in diagnosis. Instead of Jaundice, diagnosed as tuberclosis; patient died.	21.4.92	Held, medical services provided for payment by hospital and member of medical profession amounts to 'service' under the CPA, 1986. Further, consumer includes, representatives of the deceased. Deficiency of service proved; complaint allowed, granted compensation and costs.

10.	A-162/1991 II (1992) CPJ 397 (NC)	Sir Ganga Ram Hospital v. D.P. Bhandari & Ors.	Deficiency in medical services by not admitting patient in intensive care unit (ICU) and delay in providing treatment; Delhi State Commission found the hospital guilty in not informing the relatives about non-availability of vacant bed in ICU.	23.4.92	Held, there was no negligence or deficiency on the part of the hospital in not transferring the patient to ICU on account of non-availability of vacant bed; appeal allowed and State Commission's order was set aside.
11.	F.A.No. 131/1991 III (1992) CPJ 25 (NC)	Consumer Education and Research Society and Anr. v. Dr. Ratilal B. Patel & Ors.	Gross negligence in treatment. State Commission, Gujarat dismissed the complaint. Appeal made against the order.	3.8.92	Appeal allowed. State Commission's order set aside and case was remanded back to Gujarat State Commission for disposal on merit.
12.	F.A. No.97/1991 I (1993) CPJ 30 (NC)	Dr. Sr. Louie & Anr. v. Smt. Kannolil Pathumma & Anr.	Negligence in treatment. Patient's child died due to mishandling of the delivery case by doctor who was not properly qualified. Child had injuries due to vacuum slip. Kerala State Commission allowed compensation Rs.2,27000 and cost Rs.3,000. Appeal made against the order.	16.11.92	Appeal partly accepted, compensation reduced to Rs.77,000 as hospital was held responsible, not the doctor.
13.	I (1992) CPR 41	Navaneethan v. Dr. Rathinaswamy and Anr.	Negligence in diagnosis and treatment; doctors did not take reasonable care & caution.	1992	Negligence not established; Complaint dismissed.
14.	F.A.No.25/1992 I (1994) CPJ 54 (NC)	A. Narain Rao v. Dr. G. Ramakrishna Reddy & Anr.	Deficiency in service; during operation patient's tongue turned black due to inflected blood transfusion with virus Hepatitis B.	5.3.93	Held, patient was suffering with hepatitis even before the surgery; appellant has made unfounded allegations against the doctor. Appeal dismissed and findings of Andhra Pradesh State Commission confirmed with costs Rs.5,000.

15.	F.A.No.205/1992 I (1992) CPJ 257 (NC)	Miss. Gurpreet Kaur (Minor) v. Dr. R.K. Bhutani	Rashness and negligence on the part of doctor in performing operation on patient's left eye; eye lost. State Commission, Delhi dismissed complaint. Appeal preferred before NC.	5.10.93	Held, negligence or lack of due care on the part of doctor not established. Complainant deliberately, put forward a false plea and suppressed material facts such as those relating to prior operation of eye; appeal dismissed.
16.	F.A.No.243 and 265/1992 II (1992) CPJ 449	Dr. Sudhanshu Bhattacharya v. B.S. Hegde	Inadequate post-operative care in an open heart operation at the Bombay Hospital, despite paying Rs.40,000 for post-operative care, waited for 2½ hours to see the doctor, when puss was oozing from chest and undue long waiting period resulted in second operation. State Commission held, doctor had charged disappropriate amount & provided deficient services thus, awarded compensation Rs.2 lakhs and costs Rs.1000. Appeal made against the order.	7.10.93	Held, there was no evidence of any deficiency in service on the part of doctor either in performing the operation or in providing treatment as no cardiac or even serious complication arose during post-operative care; appeal allowed and State Commission's order set aside.
17.	O.P.No.221/1991	Vijay H. Mankar v. Dr. Mangla Bansod & Ors.	Deficiency in medical services.	12.11.93	Case remanded to District Forum, Nagpur, for recording evidence of witnesses.
18.	O.P.52/1992 III (1993) CPJ 402 (NC)	R. Jaya Raman v. The Poona Hospital and Research Centre & Ors.	Deficiency and delay in providing treatment for heart attack.	16.11.93	Complaint found frivolous and vexatious; held, complainant had deliberately inflated the claim to Rs.10 lakh from Rs.1 lakh; complaint dismissed with costs Rs.10,000.

19	O.P.305/1993	R.P. Agarwal v. Director, PGI	Deficiency in medical services.	13.12.93	Held, payments made for getting X-ray done not sufficient consideration; complaint dismissed with costs Rs.10,000.
20.	F.A. No. 237/1992 I (1994) CPJ 147 (NC)	R Gopinathan v. Eskeycee Medical Foundation Private Ltd.	Deficiency in operation in accidental case; State Commission dismissed the complaint; appeal preferred before NC.	4.2.94	Negligence not established; complaint dismissed with costs Rs.10,000.
21.	F.A. No. 322/1992 II (1994) CPJ 73 (NC)	M. Jeeva (Jeevan Hospital) v. R. Lalitha	Negligence in providing medical treatment in caesarian delivery; child died, State Commission, Tamil Nadu found the doctor guilty. Appeal preferred before NC.	4.5.94	Appeal partly allowed; granted compensation Rs.2,00,000 and costs Rs.10,000.
22.	O.P. No.79/1993 III (1994) CPJ 124 (NC)	Smt. Suhas Mohan Haldulkar v. Secretary, Public Health Department of Maharashtra, Bombay	Deficiency in medical services; patient died.	28.7.94	Held, free services provided by govt. institution are not covered under the Act; complaint dismissed.
23.	F.A.No.312 and 451/1992 III (1994) CPJ 72 (NC)	Orissa Nursing Home & Ors. v. Smt. Anurekha Sahoo	Deficiency in inducing labour pain; child died and patient lost her ability to bear child. State Commission allowed the complaint. Appeal made against the order.	4.8.94	Deficiency not proved; complainant allowed to prosecute before the Civil Court; State Commission's order set aside which established negligence.
24	O.P. No.100/1993 III (1994) CPJ 140 (NC)	Brij Mohan v. Dr. N.H. Banka & Ors.	Negligence and deficiency in medical services in treatment for gastroenteric problem.	9.9.94	Complaint found frivolous and vexatious; held, complainant concealed the history of his heart ailment; complainant to pay Rs.10,000 each to the doctor and hospital; complaint dismissed.

25.	O.P. No. 184/1992 I (1995) CPJ 11 (NC)	Poonam Verma v. Dr. Ashwin Patel & Anr.	Deficiency in provision of medical services; doctor being homeopath prescribed allopathic medicine; patient died.	8.11.94	Negligence not established. Held, whether a person qualified in homeopathy can practice allopathy should be taken care by govt. of India (Ministry of Health) and Medical Council of India; petition dismissed.
26.	F.A. No.497/1992 I (1995) CPJ 232 (NC)	Poona Medical Foundation Ruby Hall Clinic v. Marutirao L. Titkare & Anr.	Deficiency in service in not giving hospital's records. State Commission, Maharashtra, awarded compensation Rs.10,000. Appeal made before NC.	11.1.95	Held, no negligence on the part of hospital as discharge card and slip was provided to the patients; appeal allowed.
27.	F.A. No.41/1993 II (1995) CPJ 234 (NC)	Ramji Lal v. M/s. Sarvodaya Mediical	Deficiency in medical services; 2 month old child died.	17.2.95	Held, compensation can be awarded for any loss or injury suffered by consumer due to negligence of opposite party and here negligence is not established as child died due to congenital heart disease not diarrohoea; appeal dismissed without costs.
28.	F.A. No.97/1993 II (1995) CPJ 227 (NC)	Rahul Sinha & Ors. v. Dr. Ashok Mitra & Ors.	Negligence in writing report of C.T. Scan done for cancer by radiologist. State Commission dismissed the complaint. Appeal made against the order.	9.3.95	Negligence not established on the part of radiologist. Appeal dismissed and State Commission's order confirmed.
29.	F.A. No.588/1993 I (1996) CPJ 301 (NC)	S.B. Tiwari v. Dr. G. Pranavadhyani	Deficiency in service; removal of tooth resulted in headache.	10.11.95	Deficiency in service not established; complaint dismissed

30.	F.A. No.468 & 612/1993 I (1998) CPJ 49 (NC)	Mumbai Grahak Panchayat v. Dr. (Mrs.) Rashmi B. Fadnavis & Ors.	Negligence in operation; patient died. District Forum allowed compensation but did not held anaesthetist liable. Appeal made before NC.	15.2.96	Held anaesthetist was liable as negligence on his part established; appeal allowed.
31.	F.A. No.534/1993 II (1996) CPJ 75 (NS)	Suvarna Baljekar v. Rohit Bhatt	Deficiency in treatment; medicine had adverse effect. State Commission awarded compensation. Appeal made against the order.	6.5.96	Held, no evidence were produced to show medicine had got adverse reaction; appeal allowed.
32.	F.A. No.259, 310, 321/1993 II (1996) CPJ 209 (NC)	Salagaocar Medical Research Centre & Ors. v. R.B. Raikar & Ors.	Doctor left gauze towel in operation. State Commission allowed compensation. Appeal made for cross-examination of witness.	9.5.96	Permission to cross examination of witnesses allowed and appeal disposed off.
33.	F.A. No.570/1993 II (1996) CPJ 233 (NC)	Dr. N.T., Subrahmanyam & Anr. v. Dr. B. Krishna Rao & Anr.	Negligence in medical services.	21.6.96	Held, doctor was not guilty of negligence as in a matter of opinion he made an error of judgement; appeal dismissed with costs Rs.10,000.
34.	F.A. No.600/1993 III (1996) CPJ 75 (NC)	Sau Madhuri v. Dr. Rajendra & Ors.	Negligence in operation for caesarian child; pain continued after the discharge. State Commission awarded compensation Rs.2,000. Appeal made against the order.	29.8.96	Appeal allowed, compensation enhanced to Rs.10,000 and allowed costs Rs.2000.
35	R.P. No.698 & 699/1996 I (1994) CPJ 82 (NC)	Dr. Ashok Dhawan v Surjeet Singh	Negligence in treatment; doctor gave injection without testing resulting in non-movement of arm. District Forum awarded Rs.10,000 to patient. Revision petition filed.	14.3.97	Petition disposed off, compensation reduced to Rs.5000.

36.	F.A. No.128/1994 II (1997) CPJ 14 (NC)	Tapan Kumar Nayak & Ors. v. State of Orissa & Ors.	Deficiency in service; child given vaccination; developed reaction. State Commission dismissed the complaint. Appeal made before NC.	9.4.97	Held, negligence not established on the part of doctor as no other child developed the same reaction; appeal disposed off, and State Commission's order confirmed.
37.	F.A. No.88/1994 III (1997) CPJ 81 (NC)	Md. Aslam v. Ideal Nursing Home	Deficiency in performance of emergency operation; patient died.	29.5.97	Negligence not established. Held, patient not followed the advise given by the doctor. Appeal disposed off.
38.	F.A. No.117/1994 III (1997) CPJ 41 (NC)	Kailash Kumar Sharma v. Dr. Hari Charan Mathur	Negligence in eye operation; vision not restored. State Commission dismissed the complaint. Appeal made against the order.	29.5.97	Negligence not established; appeal disposed off.
39.	F.A. No.214/1993 II (1998) CPJ 3 (NC)	Consumer Protection Council v. Dr. M. Sundaram and Anr.	Negligence in operation; cancer patient undergone operation; died. State Commission dismissed the complaint as negligence not proved. Appeal made before NC.	29.5.97	Appeal dismissed; State Commission's order confirmed.
40.	F.A. No.52/1994 III (1997) CPJ 14 (NC)	Dr. (Miss) Jasmine Patel v. Dr. R.J. Manek Shalo & Anr.	Negligence in operation; suction instrument carelessly used resulting in multiple abdominal hernia. Maharashtra, State Commission dismissed the complaint. Appeal made against the order.	30.5.97	Case remanded back to State Commission to provide opportunity to produce evidence.
41	F.A. No.86/1994 I (1998) CPJ 10 (NC)	Sethuraman Subramaniam Iyer v. Triveni Nursing Home	Negligence in operation; complainant wife suffering from sinusitis, advised minor operation; after operation died. State Commission dismissed the	30.5.97	Appeal dismissed; State Commission's order confirmed.

			complaint as no negligence proved. Appeal made against the order.		
42.	F.A. No.506/1994 I (1998) CPJ 16 (NC)	P.P. Ismail v. Mrs. K.K. Radha	Negligence in operation, leg operated; X-ray revealed presence of foreign particle inside leg. Kerala State Commission allowed compensation. Appeal made against the order.	30.5.97	Negligence established; appeal dismissed.
43.	O.P. No.292/1994 II (1997) CPJ 98 (NC)	Harjot Ahluwalia (Minor) through his parents v. M/s Spring Meadows Hospital & Ors.	Negligence in medical services, minor was given wrong injection resulting in irreparable damage to the brain.	16.6.97	Negligence proved, compensation awarded Rs.12.5 lakhs to both child and parents.
44.	F.A. No.266/1994 II (1998) CPJ 40 (NC)	Yasmin Sultana & Anr. v. Dr. Rupaben D. Patel & Anr.	Negligence in treatment, New born child died. State Commission dismissed the complaint. Appeal made against the order.	18.8.98	Negligence not established; appeal dismissed.
45.	F.A. No.612/1993 III (1998) CPJ 21 (NC)	Dr. (Mrs.) Rasmi B. Fadnavis & Anr. v. Mumbai Grahak Panchayat & Ors.	Negligence proved by National Commission; doctor made appeal before NC.	4.9.98	Negligence proved; Appeal dismissed.

46.	O. P. No. 206/1995 III (1999) CPJ 9 (NC)	Kanhaiya Kumar Singh v. M/s Park Medicare & Research Centre	Complainant minor son operated upon for appendicitis. Complications developed. Second operation performed. Even after second operation, patient continued with pain, fever and vomitting, but was discharged. Complainant took him to another doctor where he got relief.	27.5.1999	Complaint dismissed. Held, no negligence found on the part of doctors. It was further held that negligence has to be established and petitioner has not produced any evidence to show any damage to the boy attributable to the operation since operation was performed 4 years ago.
47.	F.A. No. 283/97 III (1999) CPJ 29 (NC)	Subhashish Dhar & Ors. v. Smt. Sanjukta Sengupta & Ors.	Complainant's husband was an engineer at Damodar Valley Corporation. She developed bronchial problems, consulted doctor, condition deteriorated, consulted another doctor then husband transferred, showed to another doctor That doctor refused to follow experts advice and made rude remarks.	28.7.1999	Appeal allowed. Held no medical evidence was found against the doctors. Thus, no negligence found.

			Condition deteriorated. Then, taken again to expert. Expert affirmed that proper treatment was not given. State Commission accepted the complaint. Hence appeal was made.		
48.	O. P. No. 43/93 III (1999) CPJ 53 (NC)	Tara Chand Jain v. Ganga Ram Hospital & Anr.	Complainant was operated upon for urine trouble in a private hospital. Problem of continued urine flow could not be cured. Hence complaint was made.	25.8.1999	Complaint dismissed. Held, complaint filed by complainant is devoid of merit and deserves dismissal.
49.	O. P. No. 221/92 I (2000) CPJ 37 (NC)	Vijay H. Mankar v. Dr. (Mrs) Mangla Bansod & Ors.	Complainant alleges medical negligence in a delivery where foetus died and was not taken out and the patient died.	24.11.1999	Complaint allowed. Compensation granted Rs. 2,50,000 with costs Rs. 5000. Held, Negligence on the part of the doctor was established. Further, service in case of private nursing home providing partially free treatment comes under the purview of CPA, 1986.

50.	F.A. No. 56/2000 III 2000 CPJ 32 NC	PGI, Chandigarh v. Jaspal Singh & Ors.	Mismatched blood tranfussion was given to the deceased by a doctor of PGI. State commission awarded Rs. 2,00,000 compensation. Hence appeal was made.	29.2.2000	Appeal dismissed and State commission's order confirmed.
51.	O.P. 116/91 III (2000) CPJ 18 (NC)	Smt. Kusum Sharma & Ors. v. Batra Hospital & Medical Research Centre & Ors.	Complainant's husband died in a surgical operation of adrenal tumour	30.8.2000	Complaint dismissed. Held, risks invloved in the surgery was informed and explained and the doctor has acted in accordance with accepted practice.
52.	F.A. No. 70/2000 [I (2001) CPJ 23 NC]	S.K. Iyengar v. Bombay Hospital and Medical Research Centre & Ors.	Complainant's old mother died in the hospital. Doctor had not taken her to the ICU. State Commission dismissed the complaint. Hence appeal was made.	20.12.2000	Appeal dismissed. held, no lack of care and attention on the part of nurses, doctors in treating the patient.
53.	O. P No. 182/93 [I (2001) CPJ 31 NC]	Bhajan lal Gupta & Anr. v. Mool Chand Kharati Ram Hospital & Ors.	Complainant's son was admitted for pain and non-movement of lower and upper limbs. Subsequentlythe patient	21.12.2000	Complaint allowed. Compensation granted Rs. 2 lakhs. Held, delays and lapses in not noticing

had cardiac arrest and died. Complainant alleged in ICCU oxygen tube had come late and delay of two hours in intubating the patient.	the coming out of oxygen tube which was in a way life support system are serious matter for which the hospital administrators cannot escape liability.

In *A. Narain Rao v. Dr. G. Ramakrishna Reddy & Anr.*, the appellant Shri A. Narain Rao was the complainant before the State Commission, Andhra Pradesh, Hyderabad. The complaint was filed against Dr. G. Ramakrishna Reddy, who is the Director of Jagdumba Nursing Home, Gandhi Nagar, Hyderabad. The complainant consulted the doctor (Urologist) for an ailment of his prostate gland. The doctor advised surgery and performed it. Simultaneously, blood transfusion was also done. His tongue turned black; and the complainant alleged contamination in blood. He made no enquiry about the reasons for reaction. No medicine was administered for allergic reaction. The National Commission held that the State Commission has considered every aspect of the evidence and it was only thereafter that it came to the conclusion that the complainant had failed to prove that the blood transfusion was contaminated. The State Commission vide order dated 22.6.91 dismissed the complaint. It was held by the National Commission that the tongue of the patient can turn black if there is blood reaction but not on account of any contamination in it, and confirmed the finding of the State Commission. The National Commission dismissed the complaint and granted costs Rs. 5000.

In *Miss Gurpreet Kaur (Minor) vs. Dr. R. K. Bhutani*, the complainant alleged rashness and negligence on the part of the doctor, in performing operation on her left eye which was lost. The State Commission, Delhi had dismissed the complaint as the complainant was not able to adduce evidence to prove negligence. Hence, appeal was made against the order. The National Commission concurred with the State Commission's judgement. There was no negligence or lack of due care, attention or caution on the part of the doctor in performing the operation and in administering the treatment. Further, it was manifest that the complainant had come before the Redressal Forum deliberately putting forward a false plea and also suppressing material facts such as those relating to prior operation of eye. Thus, the Commission dismissed the appeal and directed the complainant to pay costs Rs. 7500.

In the case of *R. Jaya Raman vs. The Poona Hospital and Research Centre and Ors.* the National Commission, while holding the claim of the complainant as frivolous and vexatious, remarked that the complainant has deliberately inflated the claim to Rs. 10 lacs from Rs. one lac. The Commission dismissed the complaint and imposed a fine of Rs. 10,000 the maximum under the law, on the complainant.

In *Brij Mohan vs. Dr. N.H. Banka & Ors.* the National Commission found the complaint frivolous and vexatious; dismissed the complaint with costs Rs. 10,000 each tot he doctor and hospital as it was held by the National Commission.:

"It appears that by filing the complaint, seeking to recover a compensation of Rs. 55,90,000/- from the opposite parties, the motive of the complainant is only to indulge in speculative litigation taking undue advantage of the fact that no court fee is payable for institution of a complaint under the Consumer Protection Act."

Further, the Commission observed:

"there is an increasing tendency on the part of the litigant to indulge in speculative and vexatious litigation which the fora seem readily to oblige. We think such a tendency should be curbed. I, however, find that under Section 26 of the Consumer Protection Act, the Consumer Forums can impose by way of costs only a sum not exceeding Rs. 10,000/- on a complainant where the Consumer Forum finds that the complaint is frivolous or vexatious. Considering the magnitude of the compensation claimed by the complainant in the present case, the award of costs of 10,000/- would be pitifully small and would not act as deterrent against lodging of frivolous and vexatious complaints and harassment of suppliers of goods and provider of services who are otherwise not liable under the Act, the Consumer Forums should have the powers to adequately compensate such parties. Complainants who are maliciously and perhaps with a view a blackmail arranged under the Consumer Protection Act. I consider it my duty to make the above observations so that law makers may take notice of the same and take appropriate steps to ensure that the CPA is not misused."

In *Suvarna Baljekar vs. Rohit Bhatt*, the complainant was taking homeopathic medicine against payment. Since the medicine had adverse effect, the State Commission awarded compensation. Hence, appeal was preferred before the National Commission.

The National Commission held that the State Commission was not justified in granting any relief to the complainant. The complainant did not lead any evidence to show that he had suffered from the alleged ailments narrated by him in the complaint after taking the medicine prescribed by the opposite party. The complainant also did not lead any evidence to show that he took any treatment for any of the ailments narrated by him. Hence, the appeal was allowed and the appellant was granted the cost amounting to Rs. 1000.

In *Dr. N.T. Subrahmanyam & Anr. vs. Dr. B. Krishna Rao & Anr.*, husband of Smt. Rajalakshmi filed a complaint that his wife was admitted to be attended by Dr. B. K Rao for the complaint of vomiting of blood as she was suffering from jaundice. Although, endoscopy had already been done, her doctor referred her to Dr. Rao as he was a senior endoscopist. Since, she continued to vomit, she was admitted. Dr. Rao had stated that he had 22 years of experience in dealing with such acute cases and even according to the complainant, Smt. Rajalaxmi was referred to Dr. Rao as he was a senior and expert endoscopist. The National Commission found that earlier, Smt. Rajalakshmi had been treated five times in that nursing home, which clearly showed that the complainants were satisfied with the treatment. Further, Dr. Rao had adopted the method of treatment considering her condition at the time of her admission and was well satisfied with the care taken and the treatment. The National Commission held that the complainants had failed to prove that there was any negligence on the part of opposite party. Accordingly, the order of the State Commission was confirmed and appeal was dismissed with costs of Rs. 10,000.

It was further held by the National Commission that the principles regarding medical negligence are well-settled. A doctor can be held guilty of medical negligence only when he falls short of the standard of reasonable medical care.

In *R. Gopinathan vs. Eskeycee Medical Foundation Private Ltd owning Devaki Hospital & Anr.*, the complainant met with an accident and taken to the hospital. The duty doctor attended, got the x-ray done of the injured part of the right leg of the complainant. An operation was performed. His wife questioned the act of the doctor and took the complainant to another hospital where a second surgery was done by another doctor. It was alleged that the first operation was technically defective and, therefore, he could not return to normality. The State Commission, Tamil Nadu had dismissed the complaint, hence appeal was made against the order. The National Commission held that they did not find any ground to differ from the findings of the State Commission. The doctor was qualified in trauma and accident cases. Further, it also cannot be said that the technique opted by the doctor was not well-recognised. Therefore, it was difficult to held that the doctor was guilty of any negligence or deficiency in performing the operation. The National Commission while dismissing the complaint with costs Rs. 10,000, adopted the following observations made by Justice Barrie in Moore v Lersishan Group, with approval:

"When there are two genuinely responsible school of thought about the management of a clinical situation, the Courts could not do great disservice to the community or the advancement of medical service than to place to hall mark of legality upon one form of treatment."

In *Brij Mohan Kher v. Dr. N.H. Banka & Anr.*, the complainant who is a marine engineer by profession has come up with the complaint seeking to recover a compensation of Rs. 53,90,000 from the opposite parties, namely Dr. N.H. Banka and the Medical Research Centre, Bombay, by alleging that because of negligence amounting to deficiency in service in diagnosing and treating the complaint while he was an in-patient of the hospital, the complainant had suffered severe damage to his heart muscles and unable to resume his duties.

The National Commission held that there was evidence to show that complainant had tried to create evidence by changing the point of time at which he suffered myocardial attack. The National Commission further held that the motive of the complainant was only to indulge in speculative litigation taking undue advantage of the fact that no court fee is payable for institution of a case under the CPA, 1986. Thus, the National Commission held that the complainant totally failed to make out the case against the opposite parties and dismissed the petition as frivolous and vexatious. The National Commission also referred to the observations of the Supreme Court of India in *Morgan Stanley Mutual Fund vs. Kartik Dass & Ors.* Civil Appeal No. 4584 and 4587 of 1994 reported in II (1994) CPJ 7 (State Commission):

"there is an increasing tendency on the part of litigants to indulge in speculative and vexatious litigation and adventurism for which they (consumer courts) seem readily to oblige. We think such a tendency should be curbed."

The National Commission held that under Section 26 of the CPA, 1986, the Consumer Forums could impose by way of costs only a sum not exceeding Rs. 10,000 on a complainant where the Consumer Forums found that the complaint was frivolous or vexatious. Considering the magnitude of the compensation claimed by the complainant in the present case, the award of costs of Rs. 10,000 would be pitifully small and would not act as a deterrent against lodging of frivolous and vexatious complaints and harassment of providers of services who are otherwise not liable under the Act. The National Commission further held that the Consumer Forums should discourage such false and vexatious complaints being lodged before the Consumer Forums with a view to harassing and blackmailing those who supply the goods and provide services to the community. Thus, the National Commission while dismissing the complaint held that it would be reasonable in this case to direct that complainant should pay a sum of Rs. 10,000 by way of costs to O.P. No. 1 and a further sum of Rs. 10,000 to O.P. No. 2.

Cases relating to reduction of compensation: The National Commission also reduced the amount of compensation awarded by the State Commission in some cases. Two such cases are detailed below:

In *Dr. Sr. Louie & Anr. vs. Smt. Kanolil Pathymma and Anr.*, the complainant alleged that the doctor had misled the patients by putting an M.D. Degree though she did not possess the same. The patient died after delivering a child. The Kerala State Commission allowed compensation of Rs. 2,27,000. The doctor appealed before the National Commission. The National Commission partly accepted the appeal as the hospital was held responsible for the negligent act. The National Commission reduced the compensation payable to the victim from Rs. 2,27,000 to Rs. 77,000 and Rs. 2,000 as costs.

In *Dr. Ashok Dhawan vs. Surjeet Singh*, the doctor administered an injection to the patient. Surjeet Singh, without proper test, resulting in non-movement of his arm. The District Forum, Karnal and later, the Haryana State Commission ordered Rs. 10,000 as compensation. The National Commission held that there was no record which could throw light as to how much amount had been spent. In National Commission's opinion, Rs. 10,000 seemed to be on higher side and the amount of compensation was reduced to Rs. 5,000.

Case examining the scope of 'service': In the case of *M/s Cosmopolitan Hospital and Anr. v. Smt. Vasantha P. Nair* and *M/s Cosmopolitan Hospitals and Anr. vs. Smt. V.P. Shantha and Ors.* the National Commission examined the scope and definition of the term 'service' as defined under Section 2(1)(o) of the CPA, besides discussing the characteristics of the services rendered by professionals like medical professionals. The National Commission also defined the scope of the expression 'consumer of health services' to mean that patients as well as their legal heirs are to be included under 'consumer' as defined under the Act.

Case examining the fees charged by the doctor: In *Dr. Sudhanshu Bhattacharya vs. B. S. Hegde*, the complainant underwent an open heart operation in Bombay Hospital. The complainant alleged that the doctor did not provide adequate post-operative care and puss was oozing from his chest. He further, alleged that he waited for 2 1/2 hours and yet when no doctor attended him he was compelled to seek treatment from two other doctors, who performed a second operation.

The complainant alleged that despite paying Rs. 40,000 for post-operative care, the doctor did not provide him requisite care and attention, i.e., no reasonable proper and satisfactory care and treatment was rendered.

The Maharashtra State Commission concluded that the doctor had charged 'disproportionate' amount and provided deficient services and there were evidence to show that. The doctor was held guilty of gross negligence. The State Commission awarded Rs. 2,00,000 as compensation and Rs. 10,000 as costs and also allowed refund of Rs. 40,000 paid by complainant. Appeal was preferred before the National Commission.

The National Commission allowed the appeal and set aside the order of the State Commission as there was no evidence to show any deficiency in service on the part of opposite party either in performing the operation or in providing treatment as no cardiac or even serious complication arose during post-operative care. The National Commission the concurred with the observation made by the State Commission, "How much to charge as fee for medical services is the choice of the medical practitioner even though it may appear to be unreasonable and unjustifiable.' It was concluded that a doctor has the absolute right to decide which patient he would examine and even out of turn, depending upon the condition of the patient. There is nothing improper or unreasonable if the doctor gives precedence to a patient.

In regard to fees, the National Commission observed:

'How much to charge a fee for medical service is the choice of the medical practitioner even though it may appear to be excessive, unreasonable and unjustified ? Once the patient agrees to pay the fees even though under compelling circumstances, it will not be proper to order the refund of the amount.'

It is clear from the observation that the National Commission, even if it feels that fees charged are exorbitant, do not seem it proper to interfere in the matter of amount of fees charged by the doctors.

Case of gross negligence in provision of medical services: In *M. Jeeva vs. R. Lalitha*, M. Jeeva was running a hospital under the banner, Jeevan Hospital, Trichy. She went about declaring that she was a qualified doctor, whereas she was only a mid-wife. The complainant availed of medical services for delivery of her second child. The complainant was admitted and underwent an operation. The case got complicated and there was prolonged labour pain and a dad male child was delivered. Her uterus was also removed. The State Commission allowed compensation. Hence appeal was made by the opposite party against the State Commission's order.

The National Commission held that the appellant undertook the task which she know or ought to have known that she was not qualified to perform. Therefore, she is fully responsible for the harm which happened to the complainant and the child. The National Commission upheld the findings of the State Commission that appellant acted rashly, recklessly with culpable negligence. Thus, appeal was partly allowed and the total amount of compensation payable by appellant to complainant was reduced from Rs. 250000 to Rs. 2 lacs and Rs. 10,000 as costs as it would sufficiently compensate the complainant for the prolonged labour pain.

In *Ramanand B. Raikar v. Salgaonkar Medical Research Centre and Anr.* the National Commission observed:

"it is abundantly established from the material on record that 'gauze tower' was left in stomach cavity of complainant while performing the operation. We, therefore, are firmly of the view that there has been negligence on the part of the opposite party. No gauze towel could have remained in the abdominal cavity of complainant, if opposite parties acted with ordinary skill and with reasonable care."

In *Sau Madhduri v. Dr. Rajendra & Ors.*, the complainant was underwent a caesarean operation. After operation at Amaravati, she had pain in abdomen and continued to have pain even, after she was discharged. Upon examination, a pair of scissors were fund interests he abdomen. She was again operated and the pair of scissors were removed. The Maharashtra State Commission awarded Rs 2000 as compensation and Rs. 29,175 for further treatment. The National Commission held that compensation of Rs. 2000 was on lower side and increased it Rs. 10,000.

In *Mumbai Grahak Panchayat v. Dr. Mrs. Rashmi B. Fadnavis & Ors.*, the husband of deceased Mrs. Meena Pilankar filed complaint alleging that the deceased had died due to negligence of the doctor who was attached to Jeewan Vikas Kendra in Mumbai. On the basis of records, the Maharashtra State Commission held that death was due to negligence (due to lack or ordinary care and skill which a doctor should have exhibited under the circumstances) and awarded compensation. Death was caused because of negligence on the part of the anaesthetist. It has to be added that in this case the anaesthetist was not an employee of the hospital - his services were hired for this case.

The National Commission held that the anaesthetist who participated in the process of delivery of medical services to the beneficiary was as much liable as the main surgeon. Even if the services of the anaesthetist was hired by the doctor, the patient was beneficiary of medical services, which means that the patients is a consumer of that service.

In *P.P. Ismail v. Mrs. K.K. Radha*, the complainant, K. K

Radha's leg was operated and put under plaster by the doctor at the hospital. Later, x-ray revealed the presence of foreign particles inside the leg. A second opinion was taken and emergency operation was done to save her leg and plastered again. The complainant remained in the hospital for 25 days. The Kerala State Commission allowed the complaint and awarded damages. Therefore appeal was preferred before the National Commission. The National Commission held that the State Commission rightly held the opposite party liable.

In *Spring meadows Hospital and Anr. v. Harjot Ahluwalia*, the parents filed a complaint on behalf of a minor and alleged that the child on account of negligent and deficiency on the part of hospital authorities doctors and nurses suffered irreparable damages and his brain was damaged. The child could survive only as a mere vegetative. The National Commission awarded Rs. 12.5 lacs as compensation to the minor and Rs. 5 lacs to the parents. The cause of brain damage was high doses of injection lariago. Appeal was preferred before the Supreme Court.

The Supreme Court held that both child (minor) and his parents were Consumers under section 2(1)(d) of the CP Act and the National Commission was fully justified in awarded compensation to both child and parents for metal agony and loss suffered by each of them.

Cases relating to service provided free of charge by government hospitals : Not covered under the Act: Complaints against government hospitals are found to be getting dismissed by the National Commission from the very beginning. In *Consumer Unity and Trust Society vs. State of Rajasthan & Ors.* the complainant underwent tubectomy operation at a government hospital. Complications developed and she became physically invalid. The State Commission, Jaipur held that free services are not covered under the Act. Hence, appeal was preferred before the National Commission. The National Commission rejected the appeal and held:

"Persons who avail the facilities of medical treatment in

government hospitals are not consumers and the said service cannot be regarded as service hired for consideration."

In *R.P. Agarwal vs. Director, PGI*, the Commission held that some payments made for getting x-ray done was not sufficient consideration to come under the purview of the Act.

In *Smt. Suhas Mohan Haldulkar and Ors. vs. Secretary, Public Health Department, Govt. of Maharashtra, Bombay & Ors.*, the complainant alleged that the treatment administered to her husband at the hospital suffered from deficiency and negligence as a consequence of which her husband died. The National Commission held that the aforesaid hospital, i.e. J.J. Hospital was a government run hospital where patients were treated wholly free of charge. Such being the case the service rendered by the hospital would not constitute service under the CPA, 1986 as had been laid down by this Commission in *Consumer Unity and Trust Society, Jaipur vs. State of Rajasthan*, First Appeal No. 2 of 1989 decided in December 12, 1989. Thus, the National Commission dismissed the complaint.

Cases relating to seeking of expert opinion: The National Commission do seek expert opinion wherever felt necessary. Even in civil and criminal cases, expert advice is taken by the Courts. In the case of *Mr. Mohd. Ishfaq vs. Jaslok Hospital and Research Centre*, the National Commission referred the matter to the Director, AIIMS for expert opinion. In this case, the complainant had become deaf allegedly after an injection was administered and due to negligence of the doctor.

In *K. Gracy Kutty v. Dr. Annamma Oommen and Anr.*, the Commission observed:

"Medical profession being a very sensitive area where problems connected with physical and mental health and life of living human beings are handled, this court has applied sufficient caution in assessing the issues and formulating the conclusions. This court has consulted authoritative publications on gynaecology and obstetrics and have given anxious considerations to the valuable expert opinions of professionally competent witnesses examined in this case and the relevant judicial pronouncements having bearing on the issues were referred t in deciding whether the opposite parties have applied the required degree of skill and competence and followed the accepted medical practice in this instance."

In *R. Gopinath v. Eskaycee medical Foundation and Anr.* the National Commission observed that since this complaint involves complicated questions of law and facts requiring detailed investigations, elaborate and voluminous evidence which the Consumer Forums should not entertain the complainant must be directed to seek remedy in the court of ordinary civil jurisdiction.

In *N. C. Sarin vs. Moolchand Kharaitiram Hospital and Ors.*, Smt. Vidya Sarin, a patient was admitted to hospital with pain and died of cardiac arrest. Complainant alleged negligence on the part of the opposite party.

The Delhi State Commission held that truth would come out only as a result of thorough cross-examination of the witnesses concerned. It was not one of such cases where negligence on the part of hospital or doctors was so palpable that it could be called gross negligence. The Commission was not expected to undertake such an enquiry. Thus, the complaint was disposed of leaving it open to the complainant to have his remedy in the Civil Court.

However, this is not an inviolable rule. The National Commission has itself held in *Abdul Sukur v. State of Orissa.*

"the mere fact that witness may have to be examined and their cross-examination may also be necessary, is not by itself a valid ground for refusing adjudication of the disputes before the Redressal Forums constituted under the Consumer Protection Act. It is also to be remembered from the very purpose for which the statute has been enacted is to provide a cheap and remedy to aggrieved consumers by way of an alternative to the time consuming and expensive process of civil litigation. The statute thus, clearly contemplates that the Redressal Forums constituted under it are to decide cases filed before them after taking such oral and documentary evidence on the circumstance of any given case may require. If jurisdiction is declined by the special Redressal Forums set up under the Act in all such cases on the mere ground that examination and cross-examination of witnesses would be necessary it would amount to unjust denial of the benefits of the Act to the aggrieved consumer by erroneous addiction of its jurisdiction by the Forums."

In the case of *Poonam Verma vs. Dr. Ashwin Patel & Anr.*, where the doctor of homeopathy treated Poonam Verma in a nursing home by prescribing allopathic medicines and in the end she died. The National Commission dismissed the complaint and held that whether a person qualified in homeopathy can practice allopathy should be taken care by the government of India, Ministry of health and Medical Council of India. However, while deciding the appeal, the Supreme Court held that a person who did not have the knowledge of a particular system of medicine was a quack. Where a person was guilty of negligence, no further proof was needed. The doctor having practised allopathy, without being qualified in this system was guilty of negligence, so appeal against him was allowed and compensation was allowed as claimed (Rs. 3 lacs).

Cases where opportunity given to produce evidence: In *Sunil Blood Bank and Transfusion Centre vs. Shri Naresh Kumar and Anr.*, the complainant alleged transfusion of contaminated blood with Hepatitis B virus. The State Commission Delhi allowed the complaint and granted compensation of Rs. 20,000 In the appeal, the National Commission remanded the case back to the State Commission to dispose of afresh after giving adequate opportunity to both parties to adduce oral and documentary evidence.

The National Commission also took into consideration the place of residence of the witnesses. In case of *Vijay H. Mankar vs. Dr. (Mrs) Manala Bansod and Ors.*, the National Commission remanded the case to the District Consumer Dispute Redressal Forum, Nagpur, for recording of evidences of various witnesses since witnesses of both the parties resided at Nagpur.

In *Dr. (Mrs) Jamine Patel vs. Dr. R.J. Manek Shah & Anr.*, the complainant got operated and suffered complications, and alleged gross negligence. The Maharashtra State Commission dismissed the complaint. Hence, appeal was preferred before the National Commission. The National Commission held that the State Commission's order did not adequately deal with the allegations of the complainant. Therefore the case was remanded back to the State Commission for giving an opportunity to the complainant to produce evidence.

In *Salgaocar Medical Research Centre & Ors. vs. R.B. Raikar & Ors.*, the complainant alleged that the doctor did not use reasonable skill and diligence in operating on him as the doctor had left gauze towel in the patient's stomach. Therefore, he suffered physical agony and had to undergo prolonged and expensive treatment and had also to undergo another operation in Jaslok Hospital where the towel was removed from the stomach. The opposite party moved an application for cross-examination of witnesses. This application was not allowed by the State Commission, which had allowed compensation. hence, appeal was made against the State Commission.

The National Commission held that the view and procedure adopted by the State Commission, not giving permission to cross-examine the witnesses of the complainants on the ground that under Section 13(4) (iii) of the Consumer Protection Act 1986, the reception of evidence on affidavit was legal and it further remarked that the affidavit was sufficient to establish the negligence on the part of opposite party, were not appreciable. It was further held that when a party insisted that he wanted to cross-examine the deponent of the affidavit, natural justice required that permission be given. Thus, the State Commission should allow the parties to cross-examine such witnesses whose affidavit have been filed and whom the other parties wish to cross-examine.

Cases in which negligence not established in the provision of medical services : In *Smt. Renu Jain & Ors., vs. Escorts Heart*

Institute and Research Centre, the husband of the complainant was admitted in hospital for coronary by-pass surgery. After the operation, complications developed and he died. She alleged deficiency on the part of the hospital in treating the patient and in taking post-operative care whereby he got infection in the leg.

The National Commission dismissed the complaint as no negligence was proved in diagnosis and in providing treatment to the patient in the hospital as the cause of death was brainstem haemorrhage, not the infection in the leg.

The National Commission in the case of *Sir Ganga Ram Hospital v D. P. Bhandari* while setting aside the appeal held that negligence or deficiency could not be attributed to the hospital merely on the ground that the hospital did not inform the relatives of the patient that they might if they chose so, remove the patient to some other hospital in view of the non-availability of any bed in the intensive care unit.

In *S.B. Tiwari v. Dr. G. Pranavadhyani*, the complainant went to the doctor for removal of tooth. He suffered headache. The State Commission dismissed the complaint on the basis of evidence produced by both the parties. The State Commission came to the conclusion that there was no deficiency of service on the part of the opposite party as the opposite party had taken the blood pressure and the complainant had not adduced adequate evidence to show that he was sent back without finding the reason for his bleeding. Further, there was no evidence to link the headache with the extraction, but headache was due to his hypertension. Thus, National Commission confirmed the order of the State Commission and the appeal was dismissed.

In *Consumer Protection Council, Tamil Nadu and Ors. vs. Dr. M. Sundaram and Anr.*, Mrs. Rajalakshmi was admitted in Dr. Sundaram's nursing home on August 1, 1991 with the complaint of vomiting. Dr. Sundaram suspected cancer and hence took a bone marrow sample for pathological testing. The testing was done by Dr. S. Anuradha who gave a report on 2.8.91. Without referring to cancer specialist Dr Sundaram started treatment with

5 doses of injection because of which she had kidney failure and died. The Tamil Nadu State Commission had dismissed the appeal as 15.2.93. It was noticed that any consultant physician of the standing of Dr. Sundaram would have not have delayed the chemotherapy when repeated examination of bone marrow yielded the report of cancer. Moreover, Dr. Anuradha was highly qualified, holding an M.D. degree in that speciality. The National Commission confirmed the findings of the State Commission and dismissed the appeal.

In *S.S. Iyer v. Triveni Nursing Home*, the complainant's wife suffering from sinusitis was advised a minor operation. Expenses and risks were inquired about and the patient got operated upon. The lady died due to heart failure. These dismissed the complaint, since from the operation notes, it appeared that necessary efforts were made to save her. Hence, appeal was preferred before the National Commission. The National Commission held that the State Commission had rightly relied upon operation notices and there was no negligence on the part of the doctor. It was further held that the State Commission had rightly analysed and appreciated the material placed on records. From the records, it appeared that necessary medicines were given and other possible efforts were made to revive her.

In *Poona Medical Foundation, Ruby Hall Clinic vs. Marutirao L. Tikare & Anr.*, appeal was made by Poona Medical Foundation which was running a hospital by name, Ruby hall Clinic. The complainant was admitted for back pain, operated for ulcer and appendix. He got discharged. After 3 years, he filed a complaint before the State Commission, Maharashtra alleging that there was deficiency in service in providing treatment. He also alleged that medical papers of hospital were not given to him.

The National Commission held that there was no question of negligence on the part of the appellant with regard to failure in supplying to the complainant copies of hospital records pertaining to surgical operation. The National Commission allowed the appeal.

In *Ramjilal vs. M/s Sarvodaya Medical*, a two month old baby fell ill and the doctor prescribed medicine. Medicines were purchased from M/s Sarvodaya Medical, Jaipur and given to the child. The child died. The National Commission held that the cause of death was Cyanotic congenital heart disease with congestive heart failure, and not diarrhoea, for which the medicine was given. Hence, appeal was dismissed. The National Commission further held that compensation can be awarded for any loss or injury suffered by consumer due to negligence of opposite party. In this case, negligence of opposite party was not the cause of death.

In *Rahul Sinha & Ors. vs. Dr. Ashok Mitra & Ors.*, Smt. Sushma Sinha having a medical history of cancer was operated for removal of uterine tumours. Treatment for cancer was given and again C.T. Scan was done by Dr. Ashok Mitra (Radiologist). The complainant alleged that report was not correct. The National Commission held that after carefully going through the report in which the radiologist had written that compared to previous C.T. Scan, the lesion showed no change in size and extent. Thus, no negligence was established on the part of the radiologist. Hence, appeal was dismissed.

In *Tapan Kumar Nayak & Ors. vs. State of Orissa & Ors.*, the child of the complainant was given DPT injection, with the result that he developed serious reaction. None of the other children who had been vaccinated out of the same batch of vaccine had suffered any complication of the same kind. The State Commission had dismissed the complaint. Hence, appeal was made against that order. The National Commission confirmed the order passed by the State Commission and dismissed the complaint on the ground that no negligence had been made.

In *M.D. Aslam vs. Ideal Nursing Home & Ors.*, the patient approached the doctor in the nursing home for operation for removal of uterus and ovaries and the operation was performed. Patient was advised to avoid rich food. In spite of advise, patient had been taking rich food resulting in soakage of wound.

Emergency operation was done for closure of the abdomen. The complainant developed cardiac unrest and died. The State Commission dismissed the complaint. Hence, appeal was preferred before the National Commission. The Commission held that State Commission was correct in its findings that there was no negligence on the part of doctors and nursing home. On record, it appeared that the patient was not following the advise the doctors. Hence, appeal was dismissed.

In *Kailash Kumar Sharma vs. Dr. Hari Charan Mathur*, the complainant got his eye operated, however, vision was not restored. The State Commission dismissed the complaint. Hence, appeal was made against their order. The National Commission confirmed the order of the State Commission and dismissed the complaint as no evidence or documents had been produced to establish negligence.

In *Yasmin Sultana & Anr. vs. Dr. Ruaben Patel & Anr.*, the complainant delivered a male child who died in the hospital. The State Commission dismissed the complaint as complainant had failed to establish the negligence. Hence, appeal was made before the National Commission. The Commission dismissed the appeal and confirmed the order of the State Commission as the State Commission had taken into considerations all relevant materials and evidence.

It would appear that the National Commission trends to apply stringent tests for the establishment of any deficiency or negligence on the part of services rendered by medical professionals. The burden of proof is put on the complainant, as would appear from the above cases, fail to produce any significant expert medical opinion in their favour.

Approach to the State Commissions: A summary of the major cases decided by the State Commission of various States in India, relating to deficiency in medical services since their inception till January 31, 2001, is shown in Table 3.10.

The cases reviewed in the foregoing indicate that out of a total of 225 cases decided by various State Commissions, 54 (24 per

Table 3.10

Summary of Major Cases relating to Deficiency in Medical Services Decided by Various State Commissions

(Since inception till January 31, 2001)

Sr. No.	Complaint/ Appeal No./Source	Case Title	Decided by the State Commission	Basis of Complaint	Final Order	
					Date	Summary
1.	C.C.No.1/1988	Consumer Unity and Trust Society, Jaipur v. The Secretary, Medical and Health Department, Jaipur and Director, Medical & Health Department (Family Welfare), Jaipur	Rajasthan SCDRC, Jaipur	Negligence in performing operation and carelessness in post-operative care in a govt. hospital.	3.1.89	Held, complainant has not hired services of govt. hospital for 'consideration'. Hence, not a consumer within the meaning of the Act and complaint cannot be maintainable; complaint rejected.
2.	C.C. No.3/1989	Hanuman Prasad Darban v. DR. C.S. Sharma	Rajasthan SCDRC, Jaipur	Negligence and carelessness in providing treatment in government hospital. Patient's leg had been amputated.	20.6.89	Held, complainant is not consumer within the meaning of section 2(1)(d) of the CPA as services rendered by government hospitals free of charge are not covered under the Act; complaint rejected.
3.	A-2/1990 II (1991) CPJ 503	R.B. Seth Jessa Ram & Ors. v. Sushma	Delhi SCDRC, New Delhi	Refund of tubectomy operation fee as operation was done under the Family Welfare Scheme of Government of India.	5.4.90	Complaint allowed; State Commission allowed the refund.
4.	C.C.No.44/1990 I (1992)/CPJ 182	A.K. Pias v. Kanthas Hospital	Kerala SCDRC	Negligence in treatment of snake bite, patient died	23.1.91	Held, nothing found on records to show negligence of the doctor; complaint dismissed

5.	C-3/1990 I (1991) CPJ 309	Ram Kali & Ors. v. Delhi Administration & Ors.	Delhi SCDRC, New Delhi	Deficiency in sterilization operation in ESI hospital. Operation done free of charge, women got pregnant .	25.2.91	Held, services rendered without consideration not covered under the Act; complaint dismissed.
6.	C.No.C-91/1990 I (1991) CPJ 645	Haresh Kumar v. Sunil Blood Bank & Ors.	Delhi SCDRC, New Delhi	Deficiency in services; supplied contaminated blood with virus Hepatitis 'B'.	27.3.91	Complaint allowed and granted compensation Rs.20000.
7.	C.D. No.6/1990	A. Narain Rao v. Dr. G. Ramakrishan Reddy & Ors.	SCDRC, Andhra Pradesh	Deficiency in blood transfusion, blood contaminated with virus hepatitis `B'.	22.6.91	Held, complainant was suffering from hepatitis before the transfusion of blood; complaint dismissed with costs.
8.	A.No.48/1991 II (1992) CPJ 850	Sai Medical Stores v. R.D. Gupta	Madhya Pradesh SCDRC, Bhopal	Deficiency in service; complainant purchased medicine from medical store as per doctors prescription. Medical store gave another tablets. District Forum, Gwalior awarded compensation Rs.5,000. Appeal made against the order.	26.10.91	Held, while dispensing medicine store should be strictly vigilant but wrong supply of medicine has only prolonged the recovery; appeal allowed and granted compensation Rs.2,000.
9.	II (1991) CPJ 460.	Mappooyan v. Dr. Premavathy Elango	Tamil Nadu SCDRC	Negligence in treatment ; wife of complainant took treatment from a family friend free of charge: injection given; died.	31.12.91	Held, patient was not a consumer as treatment was given free of charge, thus complaint was outside the purview of the Act; complaint dismissed.

10.	A.No. 114/1991 I (1991) CPJ 645	Shri Naresh Kumar & Anr. v. Sunil Blood Bank and Transfusion Centre	Delhi SCDRC, New Delhi	Negligence in treatment; transfusion of contaminated blood by virus Hepatitis `B'.	10.1.92	Complaint allowed and granted compensation Rs.20000.
11.	C.No.C-135/1990 I (1992) CPJ 257	Miss Gurpreet Kaur (Minor) v. Dr. R.K. Bhutani	Delhi SCDRC, New Delhi	Negligence in operation; left eye lost.	6.3.92	Negligence not established; complaint dismissed.
12.	O.P. No.199/1991	R. Gopinathan v. Eskeycee Medical Foundation Private Ltd. owning Devaki Hospital	SCDRC, Tamil Nadu	Deficiency in treatment; operation was defective.	10.4.92	Deficiency not proved; complaint dismissed.
13.	C.C.No.47/1990	Anuradha Sahoo v. Orissa Nursing Home & Anr.	Orissa SCDRC	Deficiency on the part of Nursing Home in providing treatment	6.7.92	Held, continuing such a patient in nursing home was a deficiency in service; complaint allowed and granted compensation Rs.1 lakh.
14.	O.P. No.183/1991	R. Lalitha v. M. Zeeva	Tamil Nadu SCDRC, Madras	Negligence in providing treatment in caesarian delivery; child died.	10.7.92	Complaint allowed and granted compensation Rs.250000 & admission charges Rs.2000

15.	C.C.No.31/1992	Sachin Aggarwal Alias Vicky v. Dr. Ashok Arora	Haryana SCDRC, Chandigarh	Negligence in operation of fractured bone as a result three more operations were done. Child of 13 years had been virtually invalidated.	29.10.92	Negligence not proved against doctor. Held, ease and inexpensive nature of the consumer jurisdiction should not be allowed to become a vicious weapon, in the hands of unscrupulous patients to harass the medical doctors without good and adequate cause; complaint dismissed with costs Rs.2000..
16.	C. No. 22/1992 II (1993) CPJ 1038	Vaghri Gopalbhai Maheshvhari v. Parmar Navalben Balabhai & Anr.	Gujrat SCDRC, Ahmedabad	Negligence in treatment in a case of twin delivery where only one child was delivered and discharged. Patient died on the way to another hospital.	12.11.92	Negligence not established; complaint dismissed..
17.	C.C. No. 72/1991 I (1995) CPJ 42	Chanchal Oswal v. SDM Hospital and Dr. Nimish A. Shah	Rajasthan SCDRC, Jaipur	Negligence of doctor and hospital in a heart surgery where surgical gauze left in patient's body; second operation performed.	28.11.92	Held, there was no evidence to prove that during operation surgical gauze was left in chest which was removed in second operation; negligence not established; complaint dismissed.
18.	II (1992) CPJ 746	M. Arunachala Vadivel & Ors. v. Dr. N. Gopalakrishanan	Tamil Nadu SCDRC	Negligence in operation; patient died.	1992	Held, nothing has been left undone to patient. Negligence not found in providing treatment to patient; complaint dismissed.

19	1992 (I) CPR 77	Diwakar Konchady v. Dr. K.N. Charian	Tamil Nadu SCDRC, Madras	Negligence in operation, complainant undergone by-pass surgery; operation failed and had to continue on medicine throughout his life.	1992	Negligence not established; held, success of operation depends upon many factors; complaint dismissed.
20.	O.P. No.260/1992 II (1993) CPJ 1211	P.S. Govindarajan v. General Manager, Integral Coach Factory & Anr.	Tamil Nadu SCDRC, Madras	Negligence in treatment; complainant's wife suffered from heart attack; reached hospital, treatment given, died.	16.2.93	Negligence not established; held, best possible treatment was given; complaint dismissed.
21	C.D. Case No.36/1992 II (1993) CPJ 1209	Dipti De Sarkar v. State Authority of India Ltd. & Ors.	Orissa SCDRC, Cuttak	Negligence in treatment; deceased bitten by a cat, approached doctor; treatment given, died.	27.2.93	Held, doctor has given treatment with facilities available in the hospital. Negligence not established; complaint dismissed.
22.	Misc. P. No.908/1993 II (1994) CPJ 523	Dr. G.C. Batalia v. The Consumer Disputes Redressal Forum & Anr.	Madhya Pradesh SCDRC	Deficiency in medial services; are medical services covered under the CPA?	24.4.93	Held, medical services provided are covered under the CPA; complaint allowed.
23.	C.D. Case No. 40/1992 II (1993) CPJ 1066	Bhagabat Saran Agarwal and Anr v. State of Orissa & Ors.	Orissa SCDRC, Cuttak	Deficiency in treatment; pallet of shot gun hit eye of complainant's son; taken to govt. hospital; pellet not removed.	20.5.93	Held, pallet not removed as it may cause harm to patient; text-book supported this. Complaint dismissed.
24	C. No.165/1991 I (1994) CPJ 373	Haribhai Lagharbhai Solanki & Ors. v. Dr. Suresh Parikh	Gujrat SCDRC, Ahmadabad	Deficiency in medical service; injection given, patient died.	21.7.93	Held, no evidence produced to show death was due to treatment taken; complaint dismissed.

25.	O.P.No.41/1993 I (1994) CPJ 397	Pavitar Singh and Ors. v. State of Punjab and Ors.	Punjab SCDRC	Deficiency and negligence in performing tubectomy operation in a civil hospital; patient died.	17.8.93	Held, services provided free of charge not included in 'service' under the Act; complaint dismissed.
26.	C C.No.53/1991 II (1994) CPJ 90	Surendra Kumar Kumawat & Anr. v. Dr. (Smt.) Sunil Jain & Ors.	Rajasthan SCDRC	Negligence in diagnosing a male child in sonography; not performed DNC operation (abortion).	19.8.93	Held, not carrying out DNC operation by itself did not constitute deficiency of service; complaint dismissed.
27.	A.P.No.260/1993 O.P. 35/92 III (1994) CPJ 219	Dr. S. Venkatraman v. M. Chandrasekaran	Tamil Nadu SCDRC, Madras	Deficiency in medical service in providing treatment by voluntary Health Centre.	20.8.93	Held, service rendered free of charge is not 'service' within the meaning of Section 2(1) (o) of Act; appeal allowed.
28.	C. No.378/1991 I (1994) CPJ 361	Bhavchandbhai Lakhani v. Dr. Bhupendra D. Sagar,	Gujrat SCDRC, Ahmedabad	Deficiency in service; operation failed, bone properly not fixed.	26.8.93	Complaint allowed and granted compensation Rs.29675 and costs Rs.3000.
29.	O.P. No.96/1993 III (1994) CPJ 237	SMN Consumer Protection Council and Anr. v. Ganga Hospital and Anr.	Tamil Nadu SCDRC, Madras	Deficiency in medical service in blood transfusion.	4.10.93	Held, hospital transfused blood acting upon certificate of blood bank; complaint dismissed.
30	O P. No.869/1991 II (1994) CPJ 449	P.P. Ismail v. K.K. Radha	Kerala SCDRC	Negligence in operation; foreign particle found inside the leg after operation.	6.10.93	Negligence established; complaint allowed.

31.	A.P.No.432/1993	Kadan Karai Nadar and Ors. v. Rakkappan	Tamil Nadu SCDRC	Deficiency in giving treatment which caused disability to patient.	8.10.93	Held, no evidence to show payment of consideration, free services are not covered under the Act; complaint dismissed.
32.	C.P.No.122/1992 I (1994) CPJ 404	A.K. Hazarika v. Saraighat X-ray & Clinical Laboratory	Assam SCDRC	Deficiency in giving wrong report of x-ray.	9.10.93	Deficiency not proved; complaint dismissed.
33.	O.P.No.209/1993 I (1994) CPJ 313	S. Iqbal Khan v. The Child Trust Hospital, Madras	Tamil Nadu SCDRC, Madras	Negligence in transfusion of blood, Instead of AB positive, B positive given; child died.	20.10.93	Held, in an emergency situation, to AB group either A or B group can be given but both A & B should not be given simultaneously; negligence not establsihed; complaint dismissed.
34.	O.P.No.304/1992 I (1994) CPJ 402	Sowbhagya Prasad & Ors. v. State of Karnataka & Ors.	Karnataka SCDRC	Negligence in performing family planning operation at a camp organised by State Health Department; after the operation, third child born.	6.11.93	Held, services were not hired for consideration, thus, outside the purview of the Act; complaint dismissed.
35.	C.C.No.82/1993 II (1994) CPJ 119	Jagan Nath v. Jindal Dental and Orthopaedic Clinic of Kaithal and Anr.	Haryana SCDRC	Negligence in treatment; plate inserted by orthopaedician in patient's fore arm; got infected; took treatment at P.G.I. where prevent ampulation of arm could be prevented. Compensation claimed Rs.24 lakhs.	9.12.93	Held, mere apprehended hazard or jeopardy to life and limb was not compensatable under Sec.14 of the Act; complaint dismissed.

36.	O.P. No.63/1993	S.S. Kahlon and Anr. v. Bawa Hosital & Others III (1994) CPJ 286.	Punjab SCDRC, Chandigarh	Negligence in medical treatment.	10.1.94	Held, no evidence produced to show that any fees was charged, hence, free service not covered under the CPA; complaint dismissed.
37.	C. No. 147/1991 III (1994) CPJ 271	M.B. Gajinkar v. St. Marthas Hospital & Anr.	Karnataka SCDRC, Bangalore	Deficiency in medical service, operation done on fractured limb failed.	20.1.94	Held, doctor perfumed the operation with reasonable degree of care and caution; complaint dismissed.
38	C No. 34/1990 II (1994) CPJ 342	Consumer Education Research Society and Anr. v. Dr. Ratilal B. Patel & Ors.	Gujrat SCDRC, Ahmedabad	Negligence and deficiency in treatment.	4 2 94	Held, treatment was not non-standard; complaint dismissed.
39.	C.D. No.152/1990 III (1994) CPJ 301	Dr. G. Sarangapani v. Mr. G. Bharat	Andra Pradesh SCDRC, Hyderabad	Deficiency in medical service, District Forum established negligence; appeal made against the order.	5.3.94	Order of the District Forum set aside and case remitted to District Forum to give opportunely to both parties to produce oral or documentary evidence as no evidence was produced earlier.
40.	C. No.349/1992 I (1995) CPJ 186	Digvijaysingh A. Zala & Ors. v. Dr. Narendra T. Vani & Anr.	Gujrat SCDRC, Ahmdabad	Deficiency in medical service; patient died.	8.4.94	Negligence not established; held, deceased was advised on phone and no fees was charged; free services not covered under the Act; complaint dismissed.

41	C. No.114/1990 III (1994) CPJ 376	Mrs. K.K. Radha v. Dr. G.U. Sekhar & Anr.	Kerala SCDRC, Thiruvananthapuram	Deficiency in medical services; method of operation not proper method; patient had to undergo five more operations.	13.4.94	Complaint allowed and granted compensation Rs.2 lakhs.
42	C. NO. 107/1990 III (1994) CPJ 358	Smt. Rina Prakash v. Dr. Dechi Ganapathy & Ors.	Karnataka SCDRC Bangalore	Negligence in operation; sponge found in second operation.	10.5.94	Negligence not proved because of insufficient evidence; complaint dismissed with costs Rs.1000.
43	C.No. 280/1991 I (1995) CPJ 455	Nuruddin Kutusuddin Balati v. Dr. L.N. Vora & Anr.	Maharashtra SCDRC, Bombay	Negligence in operation; second operation done.	10.5.94	Negligence not established; complaint dismissed.
44.	C.C. No.64 & 65/1991 I (1995) CPJ 96	Jitendra Nath v. Dr. (Mrs.) Manju Geeta Mishra & Ors.	Bihar SCDRC, Patna	Negligence in medical services.	11.5.94	Held, as criminal cases were also filed before filing this complaint; as a matter of policy and principle where subject matter is subjudice before ordinary Court, a concurrent adjudication should not be conducted under the CPA, 1986, thus, the subject matter was subjudice before the High Court; complaint dismissed.

45.	C.C. No.148/1993 I (1995) CPJ 260	Raj Kumar Agarwal v. Dr. B. Mukhupadhyay	Bihar SCDRC, Patna	Negligence in operation of fracture injury; consulted another doctor.	17.5.94	Held, when there are two form of treatment, Court should not place the hall mark of legally upon one form of treatment; complaint dismissed with costs Rs.1000.
46.	O.C. No.14/1994 I (1995) CPJ 365	Subhlata v. Ghritian Medical College	Punjab SCDRC Chandigarh	Negligence in medical treatment; complainant's husband died after kidney biopsy in a government hospital.	15.6.94	Negligence not established; held, services provided free of charge by govt. hospital are not covered under the CPA; complaint dismissed.
47.	C. No.68/1991 I (1995) CPJ 220	T. Hareendran Nair v. Dr. P. Ashokan	Kerala SCDRC Thiruvananthapuram	Deficiency in blood transfusion; blood was contaminated.	19.7.94	Insufficient evidence; complaint dismissed.
48.	C.NO. 306/1992 II (1995) CPJ 159	Kanaiya Prasad G. Mishra & Anr v. Dr. (Mrs.) Tanumati G. Shah & Ors.	Gujrat SCDRC, Ahmdabad	Negligence in operation; performed on right side instead of left side.	28.7.94	Held, no evidence found to support the case; complaint dismissed.
49.	C.C. No.55/1992 I (1995) CPJ 334	Rohini Devi v. Dr. H S. Chudawat & Anr.	Rajasthan SCDRC, Jaipur	Negligence in operation for cataract; three more operations done.	18.10.94	Negligence not established; complaint dismissed.

50.	S.C. Case No.23/1994 I (1994) CPJ 453	Mukunda Lal Ganguli v. Dr. Abhijit Ghosh & Anr.	West Bengal SCDRC, Calcutta	Deficiency in providing treatment in a government hospital.	9.12.94	Held, free services rendered in government hospital are not covered under the Act; complaint dismissed.
51.	C.No. 46/1994 III (1995) CPJ 549	Ishwardas Lekhraj Ramchandani v. Dr. P.J. Buch & Anr.	Gujrat SCDRC Ahmdabad	Deficiency in treatment for facial paralysis.	12.12.94	Held, no evidence produced to prove negligence; complaint dismissed.
52.	C.No. 7/1991 III (1995) CPJ 142	Master Ashok Kumar v. Agadi Nursing Home & Anr.	Karuataka SCDRC, Bangalore	Negligence in tampering of plaster of a fractured elbow.	24.12.94	Negligence not established; complaint dismissed.
53.	C.NO. 31/1994 I (1996) CPJ 243	Aphraim Jayanand Rathod v. Dr. Shailesh Shah	Gujrat SCDRC, Ahmadabad	Negligence in operation for appendicitis; second operation performed without consent.	28.4.95	Negligence established; compensation allowed Rs.1 lakh and costs Rs.1000.
5 4.	R.No. 11/1993 I (1996) CPJ 22	Treasury Officer & Member Secretary, Pensioner Medical Fund & Ors. v. G.K. Joshi	Rajasthan SCDRC, Jaipur	District Forum held that retired employee, availing the facility of reimbursement of medical expenses by making monthly contribution while in service are not consumer under the CPA. Hence, revision petition filled before the State Commission.	3.5.95	Held, so far as the special benefits and facility of supply of free medicine to a retired government employee is concerned, the regular monthly contribution made by him constitute a consideration and thus, complaint is maintainable; revision petition dismissed.

55.	C.No. 237/1992 II (1996) CPJ 157	Consumer Protection Council & Anr. v. Parul Clinic Maternity Home and Hospital & Ors.	Gujrat SCDRC, Ahmadabad	Negligence in operation; removal of uterus along with tumour.	6.5.95	Negligence not established as consent was taken; complaint dismissed.
56	F.A. No.330/1995 II (1996) CPJ 204	Madan Mohan v. Dr. Ashwani Sood	Haryana SCDRC, Chandigarh	Deficiency in service by Ayurvedic doctor; no relief to patient. District Forum dismissed the complaint; appeal made against the order.	28.5.95	Held, doctor not found guilty; appeal dismissed.
57.	C.No. 130/1992 I (1996) CPJ 169	Amir Ali Shakir v. St. John's Medical College Hospital, Bangalore	Karnataka SCDRC, Bangalore	Delay and negligence in treatment.	14.8.95	No delay or negligence established; complaint dismissed.
58.	S.C. Case No.559/A/1994 II (1996) CPJ 135	G.K. B. Optics & ors. v. Mrs. Nina Rao	West Bengal SCDRC, Calcutta	Deficiency in medical service, eye testing done; powerful lenses prescribed; got headache. District Forum directed refund of cost, hence, appeal made against the order.	29.1.96	Order of the District Forum confirmed; appeal dismissed.
59.	I.A. No.614 A.No.736/1995 I (1997) CPJ 600	Dr. C.V. Mathew v. P. Babu	Karala SCDRC, Thiruvananthapuram	Medical negligence; no oral evidence taken only documents produced were considered by the District Forum; appeal made against the order.	26.2.96	Held, opportunities must be provided to parties to adduce evidence; appeal allowed
60	C.NO.133/1994 II (1997) CPJ 219	Altaf Amin Bhagad v. Dr. Dhansukh B. Shah	Gujrat SCDRC, Ahmedabad	Negligence in operation; patient died when operation had just commenced.	26.2.96	Held, no evidence to show that doctor had not followed standard medical practices; complaint dismissed with costs Rs.500.

61.	C.No.273/1993 I (1997) CPJ 332.	Kanaiyalal Ramanlal Trivedi & Ors. v. Dr Styanarayan Vishwakarma & Anr.	Gujrat SCDRC, Ahmedabad	Negligence in treatment; suffered toothache, treatment given, died.	8.5.96	Complaint allowed with compensation Rs.2 lakh and costs Rs.5000.
62.	C.No.249/1993 I (1997) CPJ 295	Jayantilal Govindlal Parmy v. Managing Trustee & Ors.	Gujrat SCDRC, Ahmedabad	Negligence in operation.	16.5.96	Held, no evidence produce to support the case; complaint dismissed.
63.	S.C. No.168/0/1995 II (1996) CPJ 368	Alok Kumar Chakraborty v. Dr. Gautam Biswas & Anr.	West Bengal SCDRC, Calcutta	Deficiency in medial services; patient suffered fever and abdominal pain; got treatment; expired.	4.6.96	Held, if complainant is not benefited by the system it is his misfortune, as in any treatment, it is never claimed that every person who receive treatment should be benefited by it; Complaint dismissed with costs Rs.2000.
64.	O.P. Nos.118&190/1993 III (1997) CPJ 165	Aleyamma Varghese v. Dewan Bahadur Dr. V. Varghase & Ors.	Kerala SCDRC, Thiruvananthapuram	Negligence in operation; surgical sponge left in abdomen in operation.	5.6.96	Negligence established; complaint allowed and granted compensation Rs.98,506.
65.	C.No.84/1993 I (1997) CPJ 11	Jayendra, Maganlal Padiya v. Dr. Lalit P. Trivedi & Ors.	Gujrat SCDRC, Ahmedabad	Negligence in medical services; eye sight lost due to wrong treatment.	1.7.96	Held, doctor found guilty of negligence; complaint allowed and granted compensation Rs.10000.

66.	A.No. 226&227/1996 II (1997) CPJ 445	Dr. A.S. Karthikeyan & Anr. v. T Mariyam & Ors.	Kerala SCDRC, Thiruvanathapuram	Negligence in operation; during operation child expired, District Forum awarded compensation. Appeal made against the order.	15.7.96	Held, no evidence produce to show that services were hired for consideration; hence service not under the Act; appeal allowed.
67.	C. No.C184/1993 II (1996) CPJ 418	N.C. Sarin v. Moolchand Kharaitiram Hospital & ors.	Delhi SCDRC, New Delhi	Negligence in medical services; patient died.	22.7.96	Held, negligence was not gross negligence; Consumer Forum are not expected to take such case where negligence is not so pulpable as truth came out after cross-examination of witnesses; complaint dispose off.
68.	O.P. No.52/1995 III (1997) CPJ 382	A.P. Joseph & Anr. v. Dr. Kunjannama Mathai & Anr.	Kerala SCDRC, Thiruvananthapuram	Negligence in operation.	26.7.96	Held, in case of surgery, 100 percent success can not be achieved; complaint dismissed.
69.	A. No. 72/1996 B. III (1996) CPJ 220	A.S. Nagpal & Anr. v. Kishan Lal	Punjab SCDRC, Chandigarh	Negligence in operation; lost vision in eye operation, District Forum allowed the complaint and compensation. Hence, appeal made against the order.	30.7.96	Held, no expert evidence was produced; case remanded for leading expert evidence; appeal allowed.
70.	C.No. 77 and 252/1993 III (1996) CPJ 605	Arunaben D. Kothari & Ors. v. Navdeep Clinic & Ors.	Gujrat SCDRC, Ahmedabad	Negligence in operation of right arm; during operation patient died.	5.8.96	Complaint partially allowed; granted compensation Rs.415000.

76.	C.C.NO.525/1994 III (1996) CPJ 300	Gursewak Singh v. Dr. Jaskaran Singh,	Punjab SCDRC, Chandigarh	Deficiency in treatment of fever; injection given negligently; lost leg.	30.9.96	Complaint allowed and granted compensation Rs.1.25 lakhs.
77.	C.No. 204/1993 III (1996) CPJ 441	Smt. Rohini Pritam Kabadi v. Dr. R.T. Kulkarni	Karnataka SCDRC, Bangalore	Negligence in operation; foreign body left in abdomen.	30.9.96	Complaint allowed and granted compensation Rs.2 lakh.
78.	C.No.20/1995 I (1997) CPJ 560	Manilal Nathabhai Patel & Ors. v. Dr. Tushar N. Shah	Gujrat SCDRC, Ahmedabad	Negligence in provided treatment	14.10.96	Held, no expert evidence produced; complaint dismissed.
79.	C.No. 254/1992 I (1997) CPJ 483	D.C. Bhavani Prasad v. Krishna Nursing Home	Karnataka SCDRC, Bangalore	Negligence in providing treatment; child suffering from continuous vomiting admitted to nursing home; expired.	15.10.96	Held, doctor made every possible effort to save the child; complaint dismissed.
80.	C.C. NO.389/1992 III (1996) CPJ 259	Asha Rani v. Dr. Rohit Grover & Ors.	SCDRC, Chandigarh	Negligence in eye operation, eye sight not revived; doctor refunded the expenses, complaint made for getting compensation.	17.10.96	Negligence not established; complaint dismissed.
81.	F.A. No.283/1995 III (1996) CPJ 477	Dr. K.B. Kapoor v. Phool Dev Parshad	Haryana SCDRC, Chandigarh	Doctor charged excessive fees. District Forum allowed refund. Appeal made against the order.	23.10.96	Held, doctor can fix his fees; there is no yard stick as it differ from doctor to doctor; complaint dismissed.
82.	F.A. No.660/1994 I (1998) CPJ 358	Darshni Devi v. Rajeshwar Parshad	Haryana SCDRC, Chandigarh	Deficiency in treatment of pain in arm. District Forum dismissed the complaint. Appeal made against the order.	23.10.96	Negligence not proved; appeal dismissed.

71.	C.No. 282/1993 I (1997) CPJ 103	Devendra Kantilal Nayak & Ors. v. Dr. Kalyaniben Dhruv Shah & Anr.	Gujrat SCDRC, Ahmedabad	Negligence in operation for caesarian delivery; patient died.	5.8.96	Held, post-mortem showed negligent surgical procedure; complaint allowed and granted compensation Rs.235000.
72.	C.No.77/1993 III (1997) CPJ 224	Anthony Dass A. v. Ex. Engineer, Earth Movers Divison, BEML, K.G.F. & Ors.	Karnataka SCDRC, Bangalore	Deficiency in treatment; token deduction from salary for medical facilities; took daughter for treatment and she died.	12.8.96	Held, payment of token amount for registration made cannot be classified as 'consideration' for availing such services; complaint dismissed.
73.	C.C.No.488/1993 III (1996) CPJ 112	Nihal Kaur & Ors. v. Director, Post-graduate Institute of Medical Science & Research & Ors.	SCDRC, Chandigarh	Negligence in operation; scissors found in abdomen; patient died.	23.8.96	Complaint allowed and granted compensation Rs.1.20 lakh.
74.	C.No.88/1995 I (1997) CPJ 471	Rameshbhai P. Prajapali & Anr. v. Dr. P.N. Nagpal	Gujrat SCDRC, Ahmedabad	Negligence in operation for Cataract; lost vision.	2.9.96	Held, no convincing evidence produced to support the case; complaint dismissed.
75.	O.C. No.59&64/1993 III (1996) CPJ 263	Harbhajan Singh v. Daya Nand Medical College and Hospital & Anr	Punjab SCDRC, Chandigarh	'Delay and negligence in treatment in an accidental case, patient died in the hospital.	24.9.96	Negligence not established, held, order of Motor Accident Claims Tribunal not binding on Consumer Forums; complaint dismissed.

83.	C.No.133/1993 I (1997) CPJ 503	Meghdut Gordhanbhai Thakker v. Dr. Anupama Vidhyut Bhai Desai & Anr.	Gujrat SCDRC, Ahmedabad	Negligence in treatment; patient died.	28.10.96	Negligence not established; complaint dismissed.
84.	C.No.61/1992 I (1997) CPJ 301	B. Rama Rao v. Bantiwal Sulochana Madhava Shenoy Trust (Regd.) & Ors.	Karnataka SCDRC, Bangalore	Negligence in operation.	31.10.96	Negligence not established; complaint dismissed.
85.	O.P. No.228/1993 I (1997) CPJ 96	Joseph v. Dr. Elizabeth Zachariah & Ors.	Kerala SCDRC, Thiruvananthapuram	Negligence in caesarian operation; uterus and kidney suffered permanent damage.	13.11.96	Held, no evidence produced to support the case; complaint dismissed.
86.	O.P. No.236/1993 III (1996) CPJ 534	S. Suresh Kumar v. M/s Anand Hospital & Anr.	Tamil Nadu SCDRC, Madras	Deficiency in medical services.	15.11.96	Deficiency in service not proved; complaint dismissed.
87.	C.No. 192/1993 I (1997) CPJ 238	Master P.M. Ashwin & Ors. v. Manipal Hospital, Bangalore	Karnataka SCDRC, Bangalore	Negligence in operation; in an operation for hernia both legs of the child burnt.	18.11.96	Complaint allowed with compensation Rs.5 lakhs.
88	C No.203/1993 I (1997) CPJ 266	P.N. Sudhakar Gupta v. Anugraha Vittala Nursing Home	Karnataka SCDRC, Bangalore	Negligence in treatment; girl suffering from typhoid fever, died.	18.11.96	Held, opposite party has performed his duties to the best of his ability; deficiency not found; complaint dismissed.

89	C.No.51/1992 I (1997) CPJ 525	Y.K. Rama Murthy v. Dr. L.P. Nagarajaiah	Karnataka SCDRC, Bangalore	Deficiency in giving injection	18.11.96	Deficiency not proved; Complaint dismissed.
90.	F.A. No.574/1994 II (1998) CPJ 56	Nirmala v. Dr. (Mrs.) Usha Sethi	Haryana SCDRC, Chandigarh	Deficiency in providing treatment; pregnancy terminated before maturity, no evidence to prove negligence; District Forum dismissed the complaint. Appeal made against the order.	18.11.96	Deficiency not found; appeal dismissed.
91.	A.C. No.40/1996 III (1996) CPJ 429	Master Mritunjay v. Virender Arya	SCDRC, Chandigarh	Deficiency in providing treatment; patient admitted for tumor died; complaint dismissed by District Forum for non-production of evidence, appeal for compensation made.	28.11.96	Appeal allowed; parties were directed to produce more evidence in District Forum.
92.	S.C. Case No.447/1994 I (1997) CPJ 575	Kasturi Bhattacharjee v. Sivaji Basu & Ors.	West Bengal SCDRC, Calcutta	Negligence in operation; husband died.	31.12.96	Complaint allowed.
93.	O.P. No.29/1995 II (1997) CPJ 366	C.V. Kunhi Moosa v. Moidu's Medical Care Pvt. Ltd. & Ors.	Kerala SCDRC, Thiruvanathapuram	Deficiency in treatment; after operation paralysed; given compensation to forgo his right to ask adequate compensation by coersion & compulsion.	31.12.96	Held, Consumer Forum do not entertain complaint involving fraud, coersion & compulsion, leaving the complainant to approach the Civil Court; complaint dismissed.

94.	C. No.231/1993 II (1998) CPJ 627	Praveenbhai Khubchandbhai Soni v. Dr. Rajendra R. Shah	Gujrat SCDRC, Ahmedabad	Negligence in providing treatment and care; complainant's infant son was left for treatment by doctor to a compounder; child died.	28.1.97	Complaint allowed and granted compensation Rs.1 lakh.
95.	C. No. 424/1992 III (1998) CPJ 30	Dashrath Bhai Keshabhai Nai v. Dr. Pravia Patel & Anr	Gujrat SCDRC, Ahmedabad	Negligence in operation; after operation, patient developed impotency	28.1.97	Held, evidence showed that reasonable care taken by the doctor; complaint dismissed.
96.	C No. 12/1994 III (1998) CPJ 45	Kirtilal Gelchand Sanghvi v. Medical Superintendent, Chatrabhuj Hospital & Anr.	Gujrat SCDRC. Ahmedabad	Wrong diagnosis & treatment. complainant's son died.	28.1.97	Negligence not established for non-production of evidence; complainant could not prove the case as he did not get the help from advocates; copy of Judgement sent to State Bar Council for appropriate measures; complaint dismissed.
97.	F.A. No.498/1996 I (1998) CPJ 612	Pardeep Seth & Ors. v. Dr. Ashok Sarwal & Anr.	Haryana SCDRC, Chandigarh	Deficiency in medical services; patient died during operation due to unhygenic condition of hospital. District Forum dismissed the complaint. Appeal made against the order.	29.1.97	Appeal allowed and parties were directed to appear before the District Forum.
98.	S C Case No.296/A/1995 III (1997) CPJ 249	Manju Kumar Choudhury & Anr. v. S K Ghosh	West Bengal SCDRC. Calcutta.	Demand of higher charges; complainant's brother admitted to a hospital; charges raised, District Forum held, it is not in Consumer Court's Jurisdiction. Hence, appeal made against the order.	7.2.97	Held, higher charges to be paid; appeal disposed off.

99	C. No 119/1995 II (1998) CPJ 660	Manjulaben Vinodbhai Patel v. Dr. Harshida K. Patel & Anr.	Gujrat SCDRC, Ahmedabad	Negligence in treatment, patient admitted for MTP (abortion), uterus removed without consent.	18.2.97	Held, uterus was removed to save her; complaint dismissed.
100	O.P. No.232/1993 II (1997) CPJ 177	T. Rama Rao v. Vijaya Hospital & Anr.	Tamil Nadu SCDRC, Chennai	Deficiency in service by doctor; doctor was paying rent to the hospital for using space, can hospital be held vicariously liable ?	17.3.97	Held, hospital cannot be vicariously liable, deficiency in service not proved against doctor; complaint dismissed.
101.	O.P. No.232/1993 III (1997) CPJ 50	T. Rama Rao v. Vijaya Hospital & Anr	Tamil Nadu SCDRC, Chennai	Negligence in treatments, complainant's wife got operated, complications arose, referred her to neuro-physician, after treatment died.	17.3.97	Deficiency in service not found, complaint dismissed.
102.	O. P. No.36/1995 III (1997) CPJ 432	K.K. Ummer v. Jubilee Mission Hospital Trichur & Anr.	Kerala SCDRC, Thiruvananthapuram	Negligence in operation for hernia, infection developed.	2.4.97	Deficiency not proved; Complaint dismissed.
103	C. Case No.6/1997 II (1997) CPJ 571	Parveen Sharma v Dr. Tirath Goyal & Anr.	Haryana SCDRC, Chandigarh	Deficiency in treatment in a government hospital.	4.4.97	Held, claim sought was inflated without any break-up; complaint dismissed and complainant relegated to the Civil Court.
104	A. No 575&593/1996 I (1998) CPJ	Dr. Jyothi Vivek & Ors. v. Pradeep & Ors	Kerala SCDRC. Thiruvananthapuram	Negligence in operation; lost vision in eye operation. District Forum allowed compensation Appeal made against the order.	7.4.97	Held, doctor taken utmost care; appeal allowed, order of District Forum set aside.

105.	A. No.142/1995 III (1998) CPJ 614	Kashiram Bhimarao Kamble v. Dr. Udaya Patil & Ors.	Maharashtra SCDRC, Bombay	Negligence in treatment; patient died due to drug reaction, services of specialist engaged, patient started improving; shifted to another hospital without justification. District Forum rejected the complaint. Appeal made against the order.	9.4.97	Negligence not established; appeal dismissed.
106.	O.P. No.47/1996 II (1997) CPJ 528	A.S. Mohanan v. Dr. Joseph George & Anr.	Kerala SCDRC, Thiruvananthapuram	Negligence in treatment; complaint wife expired in intensive care unit.	10.4.97	Held, no definite allegations were there for want of care; complaint dismissed.
107.	F.A. No.106/1996 II (1997) CPJ 580	Uma v. Dr. Nishu Kharbanda & Anr.	Haryana SCDRC, Chandigarh	Deficiency in sterilization operation; child born after the operation.	28.4.97	Held, such operation does not give 100 percent guarantee; complaint dismissed.
108.	S.C. Case No.581/1995 III (1997) CPJ 469	Anup Kumar Ghosh v. Dr. T.K. Biswas	West Bengal SCDRC, Calcutta	Negligence in operation; pain continued even after operation.	30.4.97	Negligence not established; evidence and medical opinion produced; complaint dismissed.
109.	O.P.No.62/1994 II (1997) CPJ 602	M. Riaz v. P.V.A. Mohandas & Anr.	Tamil Nadu SCDRC, Chennai	Negligence in operation; after operation patient suffered pain; consulted another doctor, infection suggested.	5.5.97	Negligence not established; complaint dismissed.
110.	O.P. No.5/1995 I (1998) CPJ 203	P.R. Sumangi v. Kairali Medical Centre & Anr.	Kerala SCDRC, Thiruvananthapuram	Deficiency in treatment; blood circulation stopped due to tight plaster; hand paralysed.	8.5.97	Held, negligence not proved as paralysis can be due to other reason as well; complaint dismissed.

111.	O.P. No.44/1993 III (1997) CPJ 341	Pallattu George & Anr. v. Dr. Thankam Punnoose & Anr.	Kerala SCDRC, Thiruvananthapuram	Negligence in operation; injury to urine bag during operation.	13.5.97	Negligence not established; complaint dismissed.
112.	A., No. 533 and 662/1995 I (1998) CPJ 389	Dr. S.N. Namboodiri v. Haneefa	Kerala SCDRC, Thiruvananthapuram	Negligence in treatment; patient suffering from Jaundice; no blood test conducted to diagnose; both allopathic and Ayurvedic medicine given.	14.5.97	Complaint allowed and granted compensation Rs.40000.
113.	C.D.A. No.291/1994 I (1998) CPJ 489	Dr. B. Narasaiah v. Kande Laxmaiah	Andhra Pradesh SCDRC, Hydrabad	Wrong diagnosis. District Forum allowed complaint. Appeal made against the order.	9.6.97	Negligence not established; appeal allowed.
114.	C.D. No.267/1993 III (1997) CPJ 613	Gare Devamma & Ors. v. Superintendent, Area Hospital & Anr.	Andhra Pradesh SCDRC, Hyderabad	Deficiency in treatment, husband suffered from heart attack, given treatment, died.	11.6.97	Held, no evidence produced to establish negligence as from the case sheet produced it appeared that patient was treated carefully; complaint dismissed.
115.	O.P. No.379/1993 III (1997) CPJ 242	Lakshmi Rajan v. Malar Hospital & Anr.	Tamil Nadu SCDRC, Chennai	Negligence in operation; operation performed without providing information.	13.6.97	Held, patients were prepared 2 days before the operation; complaint dismissed with costs Rs.1000.
116.	O.P. No.379/1993 III (1998) CPJ 586	Mrs. Laxmi Rajan v. Malar Hospital Ltd. & Anr.	Tamil Nadu SCDRC, Chennai	Negligence in operation; patient admitted for lump in breast, doctor negligently removed uterus, complainant had no child.	13.6.97	Complaint allowed and granted compensation Rs.2 lakh and costs Rs.2000.

117.	A.No.408/1996 II (1997) CPJ 354	Shrimati Kulwinder Kaur v. Dr. Kiranpreet Kaur & Ors.	Punjab SCDRC, Chandigarh	Negligence in operation for caesarian delivery; suffered meningitis.	16.6.97	Negligence not established; appeal dismissed.
118.	C.No. A-61/1994 III (1997) CPJ 368	A.P. Bhatnagar & Smt. Nirmala Bhatnagar v. Dr. N.K. Patnaik	Delhi SCDRC, New Delhi	Excessive fees charged.	18.6.97	Held, no law prescribes the fees to be charged from a patient; appeal dismissed with costs.
119.	A.No. 116/1996 III (1997) CPJ 611	Dr. Sharique A. Ali v. Dr. A.M. Lahari	Madhya Pradesh SCDRC, Bhopal	Negligence in providing treatment, District Forum dismissed the complaint. Appeal made against the order.	7.7.97	Negligence not established; appeal dismissed.
120.	S.C. Case No.214/o/1995 III (1997) CPJ 336	Ranjit Kumar Das v. Medical Officer, E.S.I. Hospital & Ors.	West Bengal SCDRC, Calcutta	Deficiency in medical services. Complainant's wife, holder of ESI card suffering from pain, rushed to the hospital, not admitted and died.	7.7.1997	Complaint allowed and granted compensation from hospital Rs.2 lakh and from doctor Rs.5000.
121.	O.P. No.21/1995 III (1997) CPJ 316	Biju v. Dr. K. Kunhu Mohammed & Ors.	Kerala SCDRC, Thiruvananthapuram	Wrong diagnosis.	18.7.97	Deficiency in providing service not proved; complaint dismissed.
122.	F.A. No.454/1996 III (1997) CPJ 511	Rajni Bansal v. Dr. D.C. Mittal & Ors.	Haryana SCDRC, Chandigarh	Deficiency in medical service; no evidence produced, District Forum dismissed the complaint. Appeal made against the order.	23.7.97	Held, no evidence produced to establish negligence; appeal dismissed.
123.	F.A. No.558/1995 I (1998) CPJ 413	Force v. Dr. M. Ganeswara Rao & Ors.	Andhra Pradesh SCDRC, Hyderabad	Deficiency in providing treatment. Complainant's wife suffering from cancer, not given proper treatment. District Forum allowed compensation. Appeal made for desisting to render medical services for future.	22.8.97	Held, it is beyond the scope of the Consumer Court to give such direction; appeal dismissed and granted compensation Rs.25000.

124.	F.A. No.1134/1995 III (1997) CPJ 532	Srikrishan Nursing Home v. Smt. P. Yasoda & Ors.	Andhra Pradesh SCDRC, Hyderabad	Deficiency and negligence in prescription and treatment; patient died. District Forum granted compensation of Rs.65000; appeal made against the order.	26.8.97	Held, there was no proof of negligence; appeal allowed.
125.	C.D. No.30/1990 I (1998) CPJ 110	Air Commodore Satya Narayana v. L.V. Prasad Eye Institute & Anr.	Andhra Pradesh SCDRC, Hyderabad	Negligence in cataract operation; eye sight lost.	26.8.97	Held, no evidence produced to prove negligence; complaint dismissed.
126.	C.C. No.5/1994 III (1997) CPJ 112	K.N. Lal v. R.K. Akhaury	Bihar SCDRC, Patna	Negligence in cataract operation; lost vision.	27.8.97	Gross negligence proved; complaint allowed, granted compensation Rs.555000 & cost Rs.1000.
127.	F.A. No.538/1995 III (1997) CPJ 228	Force (Society No.596/88) v. M. Ganeshwara Rao & Ors.	Andhra Pradesh SCDRC, Hyderabad	Negligence in operation; patient of cancer of cervix got operated; died. District Forum allowed compensation. Appeal made against the order.	28.8.97	Appeal dismissed; order of District Forum confirmed.
128.	O.P. No.464/1993 I (1998) CPJ 340	Tomarino Marcel D'cruz v. Management of St. Joseph's Boy's Higher Secondary School & Ors.	Tamil Nadu SCDRC, Chennai	Negligence in treatment, boy's eye injured due to accident in school, treatment given without informing parents; boy lost one eye.	12.9.97	Negligence not proved against doctors; complaint dismissed.
129.	O.P. No.221/1994 I (1998) CPJ 533	C. Anjani Kumar v. Madras Medical Mission & Anr.	Tamil Nadu SCDRC, Chennai	Negligence in operation, patient lost voice after surgery.	12.9.97	No deficiency in providing treatment established; complaint dismissed.

130.	S.C. Case No.437/A/1996 III (1997) CPJ 557	Dr. Narayan Chowdhury & Anr. v. Dr. (Mrs.) Rita Poddar & Ors.	West Bengal SCDRC, Calcutta	Negligence in operation; complainant, a doctor undergo caesarian operation and delivered a dead child, paid no fees. District Forum held, complaint not maintainable. Appeal made against the order.	16.9.97	Held, free services are not covered under the Act; appeal dismissed.
131.	A.P. No.1229/1996 I (1996) CPJ 124	V. Chitralekha v. Director and Superintendent, I.O.G. & Ors.	Tamil Nadu SCDRC, Chennai	Negligence in treatment; complainant got infection due to blood transfusion.	30.9.97	Negligence not established; appeal dismissed.
132.	C. Case No.41/1996 III (1997) CPJ 528	Baldev Singh & Anr. v. Arya Hospital-cum-Daulat Ram Memorial Medical Centre & Ors.	SCDRC, Chandigarh	Deficiency in medical services; cancer not detected after examination.	1.10.97	Held, material evidence withheld by complainant; complaint dismissed.
133.	F.A. No.676/1996 III (1998) CPJ 289	Inderjeet Singh v. Dr. P.K. Bhatia & Anr.	Haryana SCDRC, Chandigarh	Negligence in operation; got fracture in accident, undergone operation. No negligence proved. District Forum dismissed the complaint. Appeal made against the order.	28.10.97	Negligence not established; appeal dismissed.
134.	C.C. No.39/1996 I (1998) CPJ 609	Smt. Shanti & Anr. v. Post-graduate Institute of Medical Education and Research and Anr	Union Territory CDRC, Chandigarh	Negligence in operation; pregnancy after sterilization operation.	11.11.97	Held, such operation are not cent percent successful; complaint dismissed.

135.	A.No.507&579/1997 III (1997) CPJ 387	Mayo Hospital v. Sunil Tiwari	Madhya Pradesh SCDRC, Bhopal	Negligence in medical services, sample taken for biopsy, destroyed in transit. District Forum allowed compensation of Rs.20,000 and refund of charges. Appeal made against the order.	12.11.97	Held, not only deficiency but gross negligence of inhuman nature was proved; appeal dismissed.
136.	A. No.538/1997 I (1998) CPJ 476	A.M. Mathew v. The Director, Karuna Hospital & Ors.	Kerala SCDRC, Thiruvananthapuram	Negligence in treatment, paracetamol injection prescribed for minor child; child's leg paralysed.	18.11.97	Appeal allowed and granted compensation Rs.1 lakh.
137.	A.P. No.105/1997 I (1998) CPJ 181	Kharaiti Lal v. Kewal Krishan	Punjab SCDRC, Chandigarh	Negligence in treatment for abdominal pain; injection administered in artery instead of vein, fingers amputated.	27.11.97	Appeal allowed and granted compensation Rs.50000.
138.	A. No.1003/1996 I (1998) CPJ 298	Mrs. Satwant Kaur v. Dr. Kawaljit Kaur	Punjab SCDRC, Chandigarh	Negligence in operation, child delivered through caesarian operation; cotton sponge left, no evidence produced. District Forum dismissed the complaint. Appeal made against the order.	15.12.97	Held, evidence not produced to prove negligence; appeal dismissed.
139.	S.C. Case No.440/O/1995 I (1998) CPJ 336	Mrs. Lakshmi Joy Prasad v. Dr. Cameroon & Ors.	West Bengal SCDRC, Calcutta	Negligence in treatment; child suffered injury in eye in school; no special effort were made to save eye.	8.1.98	Appeal allowed and granted compensation Rs.50000.
140	R P No 11/1997 I (1998) CPJ 45	Darshan Singh Basra v Dr. Jasbir Singh & Ors	Punjab SCDRC, Chandigarh	Death due to negligence; District Forum rejected the application to summon two doctors Hence, revised petition filed.	13.1.98	Petition allowed

141.	S.C. Case NO.33/O/1995 I (1998) CPJ 377	Bhupender Nath Das v. Maharaj Ram Krishana Mission seva Pratisthan & Ors.	West Bengal SCDRC, Calcutta	Negligence in cataract operation; eye not cured, second operation done.	16.1.98	Negligence not established; held, reasonable care was taken; appeal dismissed.
142.	A. No.460/97 III (1988) CPJ 584	Gauridevi Rameshwar Singh v. Family planning Association of India & Ors.	Gujrat SCDRC, Ahmedabad	Failure of family planning operation.	19.1.98	Held, no method of sterilization is 100 per cent safe; appeal dismissed.
143.	F.A. Nos.812& 867/1996 II (1996) CPJ 205	Prem Nata Hospital v. Smt. Poonam Mangla & Anr.	Haryana SCDRC. Chandigarh	Negligence in treatment, complainant gave birth to a premature child who died. District forum granted compensation. Appeal made against the order.	5.2.98	negligence not established; appeal allowed & no compensation granted.
144.	C.C. No. 47/1996 II (1998) CPJ 102	Bhiwani Dutt v. Nehru Hospital of Post-graduate Institute of Medical Education and Research Centre & Ors.	Union Territory CDRC, Chandigarh	Negligence of surgeon in operation; Complete disabilities of left hand.	26.2.98	Complaint allowed; and granted compensation Rs.1.25 lakh and costs Rs.5000.
145.	F.A. No.449/1996 III (1998) CPJ 7	Smt. Shanti Devi v. Dr. C.K. Mittal	Haryana SCDRC, Chandigarh	Negligence in operation, hand amputated due to wrong administration of injection. District Forum dismissed the complaint. Appeal made against the order.	5.3.98	Negligence not established; appeal dismissed.

146.	F.A. Nos. 124 and 99/1997 II (1998) CPJ 239	Dr. S.B. Jain v. Smt. Munni Devi & Anr.	Haryana SCDRC, Chandigarh	Negligence in operation, lost eye. District Forum granted compensation of Rs.50,000 hence. Appeal made against the order.	20.3.98	Appeal dismissed with costs Rs.1000.
147.	F.A. No.194//1998 F.A. No.572/1998 R.P. No.58/1998 III (1998) CPJ 242	Christian Medical Centre v. A. Shajahan	Andhra Pradesh, SCDRC, Hyderabad	Negligence in treatment; operated for cataract without enquiring about diabetic condition as a result second operation was done. District Forum awarded compensation. Appeal made against the order.	2.4.98	Negligence not established; appeal & revision petition dismissed.
148.	O.C. No.30/1997 II (1998) CPJ 335	Lekhraj v. Bharat Nursing Home & Anr.	Punjab SCDRC, Chandigarh	Negligence in treatment; complainant suffered multiple fractures, gangrene developed and leg amputated.	6.4.98	Negligence not established; complaint dismissed.
149.	O.C. No.23/1997 II (1998) CPJ 265	Paramjit Kaur & Ors. v. Doaba Hospital & Anr.	Punjab SCDRC, Chandigarh	Negligence in treatment; patient died.	16.4.98	Held, no prima facie negligence was there in the case; complaint dismissed with costs Rs.5000.
150.	F.A. No.592/1997 III (1998) CPJ 352	Salinder v. Dr. Vijay Gupta & Ors.	Haryana SCDRC, Chandigarh	Deficiency in medical services, fractured patient admitted, then shifted.	24.4.98	Held, no evidence produced to established negligence; appeal dismissed.
151	C.C. No.64/1994 II (1998) CPJ 684	Ram Babu v. Dr. Anjani Kishore Prasad	Bihar SCDRC, Patna	Negligence in operation, complainant eye damaged during operation.	27.4.98	Complaint allowed and granted compensation Rs.1,90,000.

152.	C.C. No.24/1997 II (1998) CPJ 621	Satpal Pebma v. Union of India & Ors.	Union Territory CDRC, Chandigarh	Negligence in treatment, father died due to heart attack.	1.5.98	Held, father getting more than Rs.500 p m as pension so not dependent; not entitled for free treatment; complaint dismissed.
153.	C.No.45/1995 II (1998) CPJ 494	Rajiv Kumar v. Dr. V.K. Biswas & Ors.	Bihar SCDRC, Patna	Wrong diagnosis.	21.5.98	Held, doctor has took reasonable care; complaint partly allowed and token compensation of Rs.250 granted.
154.	O.C. No.40/1997 III (1998) CPJ 39	Nita Singla & Ors v. Dr. Karnail Singh	Punjab SCDRC, Chandigarh	Negligence in giving wrong medicine, died.	26.5.98	Held, treatment was not against standards; complaint dismissed.
155.	C.No.87/1992 III (1998) CPJ 66	Smt. Nirmala R. Parab & Anr. v. Dr. Kalpana Desai & Ors.	Maharashtra SCDRC, Bombay	Negligence in operation; complainant's daughter having history of miscarriage delivered baby through caesarian operation; become vegetative (mentally unfit).	1.6.98	Held, doctors done their best to treat her; complaint dismissed.
156	C.C. No.49/1996 III (1998) CPJ 128	Dr. S.L. Dhawan v. Postgraduate Medical Institute and Research Centre & Ors.	Union Territory CDRC, Chandigarh	Deficiency in providing treatment.	1.6.98	Held, no evidence produced to prove the case; complaint dismissed.
157.	O.P. No.465/1993 III (1998) CPJ 436	C. Siva Kumar v Dr. John Arthur & Anr.	Tamil Nadu SCDRC, Chennai	Negligence in operation; patient become impotent	12.8.98	Complaint allowed and granted compensation Rs.8 lakhs.

158.	C.C. No.27/1993 III (1998) CPJ 573	Shri Arun Kumar Mishra & Anr. v. Dr. Purshottam Singh	Bihar SCDRC, Patna	Negligence in treatment, patient having six months pregnancy had spontaneous abortion, due to complications two more operations done to save life; urine appendage removed without consultation.	1.9.98	Held, operation performed with standard care; complaint dismissed
159.	C.No.297/1994 III (1998) CPJ 677	Fakruddin Abbas Bharmal v. Dr. B. Das Gupta & Ors	Maharashtra SCDRC, Bombay	Negligence in providing treatment; patient operated for hernia, died.	20.10.98	Complaint allowed and granted compensation Rs.3,84,000.
160.	O.C.No.8/1996 I (1999) CPJ 578	Smt. Rajbai v. Madhya Pradesh Shasan Sachiv Lok Swasthya Avam Parivar Kalyan Vibhag & Ors.	Madhya Pradesh SCDRC, Bhopal	Negligence in operation; patient operated upon for family planning, child born.	22.12.98	Held, family planning operation cannot guarantee 100 percent success; complaint dismissed.

161.	A. N. 88/1994 II (1999) CPJ 25	Dr. Shiv Kumar Gautam v. Alima B & Ors.	Madhya Pradesh, SCDRC, Bhopal	Patient suffering from gastro-enteritis disease. Homeopathic doctor treated in allopathic system. Patient died due to negligence in treatment.	13.1.1998	Appeal dismissed with costs Rs. 5000. Held, doctor found guilty of negligence, prohibited to practice allopathy as not legally qualified. Compensation allowed of Rs. 62,000.
162.	O. P. No. 71/1996 I (2000) CPJ 115	Mrs. Saraswathi & Ors. v. M/s Vimala Hospital (P) Ltd & Anr.	Tamil Nadu, SCDRC, Chennai	Complainant having chronic duodenal ulcer got operated and died. Deceased operated inspite of low blood haemoglobin.	13.1.1998	Complaint dismissed. Held, no negligence found. No record was produced to show the cause of death of the deceased.
163.	O. P. No. 268/1993 I (1999) CRJ 581	A. Ravi v. Dr (Mrs) Usha Rani & Ors.	Tamil Nadu SCDRC, Chennai	Negligence in Family Planning operation, Patient died	24.1.1998	Complaint allowed, granted compensation of Rs. 4,00,000 with 18% p.a. interest and Rs. 2000 as cost of the proceedings.

164.	O. P. No. 90/1996 I (1999) CPJ 587	M. Chinnaiyam v. Sri Gokulam Hospital & Anr.	Tamil Nadu SCDRC, Chennai	Patient undergone hysterectomy, HIV infected blood transferred, patient died.	9.12.1998	Complaint dismissed. No deficiency proved; HIV detected after a lapse of about 1 and 1/2 year of blood transfusion; HIV transmitted from blood transfusion proved
165.	C. No. A-84/93 III (1999) CPJ 224	Dr. (Mrs) Madhu Rana v. Smt. Bimla Gupta	Delhi, SCDRC, New Delhi	Complainant undergone re-canalisation operation, both fallopian tubes blocked. Right side tube fully recanalised. Complainant did not conceive hence alleged negligence. District Forum allowed compensation of Rs. 25,000 and refund of Rs. 18,813 plus cost of Rs. 1,000. Hence appeal was made.	30.12.98	Appeal allowed. Held conception can take place if one of the two tubes is unblocked. Doctor is not responsible if complainant failed to conceive as re-canalisation operation was successfully done. Thus no negligence established.

166.	O. P. No. 71/1996 I (2000) CPJ 115	Mrs. Saraswathi & Ors. v. M/s Vimala Hospital (P) Ltd & Anr.	Tamil Nadu, SCDRC, Chennai	Complainant having chronic duodenal ulcer got operated and died. Deceased operated inspite of low blood haemoglobin.	13.1.1998	Complaint dismissed. Held, no negligence found. No record was produced to show the cause of death of the deceased.
167.	O.P. No. 396/1992 I (1999) CPJ 683	Sri C. Sankara Narayanan & Anr. v. M/s Meenakshi Mission Hospital and Research Centre and Anr.	Tamil Nadu, SCDRC, Chennai	Complaint's daughter admitted for fever, blood urea and creativine increased. Only one dialysis for 1 and 1/2 hours given. No more dialysis given. Patient died.	5.1.1999	Complaint dismissed. Held, all necessary treatment given to bring down blood urea and creativine; no deficiency in service proved.
168.	O.P. No. 140/1996 I (1999) CPJ 691	A.J. Devarajan v. Management of the Guest Hospital & Anr.	Tamil Nadu SCDRC, Chennai	Complaint's son admitted for renal failure. Excessive dialysis given which caused convulsions and died.	6.1.1999	Complaint dismissed with costs Rs. 1000 to each of the opposite parties. Held, Patient had epilepsy previously not disclosed; convulsions were not caused by excessive dialysis. no deficiency proved.

169.	A.N. 848/1997 II (1999) CPJ 152	Dr. Ravindra Kulkarni v. Bala Saheb Ganga Ram Gavade	Maharashtra, SCDRC, Mumbai,	Patient died after profuse bleeding after delivery. District Forum awarded compensation of Rs. 2,50,000. Hence appeal has made.	6.1.1999	Appeal allowed. It was a case of sudden development of shock along with marginal laceration of cervix. Patient died due to amniotic fluid embolism. Held, District Forum order set aside. No deficiency found.
170.	A. No. 2983/SC/98 III (1999) CPJ 304	Wahid Khan v. Dr. Mohd. Abdul	Uttar Pradesh, SCDRC, Lucknow	Complainant's son suffering from blood cancer. Doctor could not diagnose for 40 days. Blood report not produced.	14.1.1999	Appeal dismissed. Held, in the absence of blood report, it cannot be said that the son is suffering from blood cancer. Hence no negligence was found.
171.	O. P. No. 294/1993 I (1999) CPJ 666	Mr. S. Ramanujam v. Dr. C. P.Sreekumar	Tamil Nadu, SCDRC Chennai	Negligence in treatment and selection of wrong mode of operation in an accidental case of hairline fracture. Patient had to undergo a major hip-replacement operation and still unable to	21.1.1999	Complaint dismissed; Widening of fracture due to mishandling was not proved. No deficiency or negligence proved.

				walk properly.		
172.	A.N. 1020/97 I (2001) CPJ 532	Sunita Rani v. Dr. Ketaki Garg	Punjab, SCDRC, Chandigarh	Patient underwent abortion. Some pieces of unborn child remained in the womb. Child born after abortion. District Forum dismissed the complaint Hence, appeal was made.	29.1.1999	Appeal dismissed. Held complainant's case was of rupture tubal pregnancy and two-three ulcer perforated the intestine which were removed. Further held that patient would have died in case operation had not been performed. Thus, no negligence established.
173.	A. N. 342/98 II (2000) CPJ 180	Dr. Ranjit Singh Buttar v. Sewa Singh	Punjab, SCDRC, Chandigarh	Complainant's son suffering from diarrhoea treated by doctor and died.	8.2.1999	Appeal allowed. Held, no negligence was found. No post mortem on the dead body of patient was got conducted to know the actual cause of death.
174.	C. No. 673/1992 II (1999) CPJ 165	Chandra Sagar D. Rajput & Anr. v. Dr. Dinesh J Shah	Maharashtra, SCDRC, Mumbai	False medical certificate was issued showing VDRL test as positive for 'Titra 1.8' which means either of spouses suffering from	11.2.1999	Complaint disposed off. Serious deficiency in service found. Allowed compensation of Rs. 50,000 and costs Rs. 10,000 plus 18% interest.

				Venereal disease. Then another test, previous results proved to be false.		
175.	A.N. 909/1997 II (1999) CPJ 593	Geeta Devi @ Geeta Rani v. Dr. Ketki Garg & Anr.	Punjab, SCDRC, Chandigarh	Case of missed abortion. Ultrasound not suggested at primary stage of pregnancy.	19.2.1999	Appeal dismissed. Treatment given was best under the circumstance. Held, mere fact that ultra sound not advised cannot be attributed any way to deficiency in services. Doctors can get the order published in the same newspaper where defamation article had been published - Complainant liable to pay Rs. 2000/- to both doctors by way of compensation.
176.	A.N. 505/1998 II (1999) CPJ 375	Dr. G. Murali v. Marakkal Janardhanan & Anr.	Kerala, SCDRC, Thiruvananthapuram	Complainant got fixed a denture of two front teeth. One of them broke, approached for replacement. That did not fitted properly.	4.3.1999	Appeal allowed. Held, no deficiency in service was found. Denture made by opposite party could be made suitable by grinding but complainant did not agree.

				District Forum found deficiencies and allowed compensation of Rs. 1000 and cost Rs. 5000.		
177.	A. N. 705/1998 II (1999) CPJ 60	Mrs. Meenakshi v. Dr. Surekha Sachar & Anr.	Punjab, SCDRC, Chandigarh	Negligence in performing blood transmission, blood transfusion of B-negative had been given to B-positive, Patient felt restlessness and swelling in the body.	5.3.1999	Appeal dismissed. Held, patient failed to give correct information. R.H. factor can be influenced by medicine taken by patient. Transfusion of B-negative to B-positive blood group is a recognised treatment. Negligence cannot be attributed if doctor acts in accordance with general and approved practice of medicine.
178.	OP No. 25/98 I (2001) CPJ 409	M.J. Joseph & Ors. v. Dr. P. J. John & Ors.	Kerala, SCDRC, Trivandrum	Meat piece struck in throat. It was dislodged to the stomach and discharged. Pain and vomiting then taken to another hospital	10.3.1999	Complaint dismissed. Held, method adopted in negotiating the foreign body was medically accepted. No vital sign justifying perforation noticed till the patient was discharged. Thus, no

				and underwent surgery and died.		negligence proved.
179.	O. P. No. 16/98 III (1999) CPJ 345	Bhagwan Das Arora v. Dr. Ashok Singal	Punjab, SCDRC, Chandigarh	Complainant underwent operation for removal of tumour but there was profuse bleeding. patient referred to CMC, Ludhiana, but died on the way. Forceps discovered in the remains of deceased. FIR lodged.	16.3.1999	Complaint dismissed. Held no negligence on the part of doctors. Forceps intentionally left in order to stop bleeding. Further expert evidence not produced. Complainant tried to drag the doctor in litigation liable to pay Rs. 15,000 as compensation plus costs to the doctor.
180.	CC No. 10/96 II (2000) CPJ 308	N.K. Kohli v. Bajaj Nursing Home and Ors.	Madhya Pradesh, SRDRC, Bhopal	Complainant's wife died after operation for removal of gall bladder by lapcroscopic method. Subsequently intestinal obstruction was detected.	24.3.1999	Complaint allowed with costs Rs. 5,000 and compensation of Rs. 50,000. Held Nursing Home was deficient in not issuing a discharge certificate prescribing post-operative care. Had this been done a ERCP test been advised, a precious life may probably have been saved.

181.	A. N. 1047/97 II (2000) CPJ 205	Shashi Bala v. Sushil Kumar	Punjab, SCDRC, Chandigarh	Negligence on the part of pathological lab preparing incorrect and false report. Lab given report of blood test positive for an injection. Then got sample tested at other places. Blood test come out to be negative for injection. District Forum allowed compensation of Rs. 5000 and cost Rs. 500. Hence appeal was made.	29.3.1999	Appeal dismissed with cost Rs. 500. Lab preparing false and incorrect report amounts to unfair trade practice. Held, complainant has to be compensated.
182.	O.P. No. 201/1997 II (1999) CPJ 485	S. Tharani & Ors. v. South Railway H.Q. Hosp. & Anr.	Tamil Nadu, SCDRC, Chennai	Patient a railway employee got free medical services, died.	5.4.1999	Complaint dismissed. Held, Free services are not covered under the CPA. Hence he was not a consumer under the Act.

183.	C.C. No. 132/1992 II (1999) CPJ 391	Shiv Gopal v. Dr. (Smt.) Sudha Gupta & Anr.	Uttar Pradesh, SCDRC, Lucknow	Treatment undertaken during pregnancy for tendency of abortion. Complete bed rest advised. Patient died.	7.4.1999	Complaint dismissed. Instructions of doctors not followed. Medicines to prevent abortion was given. Held, death was due to congestive heart failure, a spontaneous occurrence and it was not possible to save patients in such cases. Thus, no negligence proved.
184.	O. P. No. 23/1996 II (1999) CPJ 555	Smt. Panjali & Anr. v. Dr. (Mrs) S. Jamuna Lokanathan	Tamil, Nadu, SCDRC	Treatment given for termination of pregnancy, condition deteriorated, emergency operation performed. Uterus and damaged intestine removed.	7.4.1999	Complaint dismissed. Held, Negligence not proved as documents not proved by persons who issued them.
185.	A. N. 530/1998 II (1999) CPJ 57	Director, Mary Queen's Mission Hospital v. M.J. Jose	Kerala SCDRC, Thiruvananthapuram	Complainant had ulcer on legs, saw an eye-catching advertisement- complete cure by imported vaccine	7.4.1999	Appeal dismissed. Held unfair trade practices proved. Material facts were suppressed by Hospital and treatment prolonged. Complainant entitled to compensation of

				promised - treated for about 15 month. Ulcer did not subside. Condition aggravated requiring removal of patient to other hospital. Alleged, Treatment prolonged though ailment was incurable.		Rs. 12,000 awarded by District Forum.
186.	F.A. No. 304/1996 II (1999) CPJ 6	Dr. N. Sandhya Rani v. M. Kalpana & Anr.	Andhra Pradesh, SCDRC, Hyderabad	Pregnancy after tubectomy operation. District Forum allowed compensation. Hence appeal was made.	9.4.1999	Appeal allowed. District Forum set aside. Held, doctor had good experience in conducting such operations. Failure rate of such operation is 0.2%. Thus, doctor was not guilty of deficiency in service.
187.	C. D. No. 163/1992 II (1999) CPJ 208	Consumer Awareness & Research Society & Anr. v. Healing Touch Hospital Pvt. Ltd.	Andhra Pradesh, SCDRC, Hyderabad	Child of 1 year having fever admitted. Child Died. Opposite party delegate responsibility to junior doctor.	13.4.1999	Complaint dismissed. Held, Opposite party's presence was not necessary. Duty doctor was himself a qualified paediatrician and constantly watching child's condition. No evidence regarding

						incorrectness of diagnosis or treatment. Hence no deficiency proved.
188.	C. C. No. 401/SC/92 I (2000) CPJ 201	Naved Ahmed v. Dr. Rakesh Kacker	Uttar Pradesh, SCDRC, Lucknow	In an operation gauge was left in the stomach. Again operation was done in another hospital and gauge was taken out. Alleged negligence.	15.4.1999	Ordered accordingly. Held as the criminal case is pending in the criminal court therefore, it will be expedient in the interest of the justice to stay the proceedings of the case till criminal case is decided.
189.	C.C. No. 11/97 III (1999) CPJ 208	Kiranjeet v. Dr. Nirlep Kaur & Ors.	Union Territory of CDRC, Chandigarh	Complainant admitted for caesarean delivery. Child died. Complainant alleged negligence.	17.4.1999	Complaint dismissed. Held, foetus was already dead before surgery. Further, patient gave birth to male child after it. Thus no deficiency in service was found.
190.	A. No. 752/98 I (2000) CPJ 134	Dr. C. V. Mathew v. P. Babu & Anr.	Kerala, SCDRC, Thiruvananthapuram	Complainant admitted in connection with third pregnancy, MTP done without prescribed qualification at hospital not	24.4.1999	Appeal dismissed. Held negligence on the part of opposite party proved. Further, it was held that doctor 'fell below the standard of a reasonably competent practitioner'.

				recognised for doing it. Further possibility of incomplete evacuation not considered. District Forum allowed compensation of Rs. 10,000. Hence appeal was made.		
191.	F.A. No. 818/1997 II (1999) CPJ 420	Dr. Anumalla Satya Narayana v. K. Shankar	Andhra Pradesh, SCDRC, Hyderabad	Complainant admitted for pain in leg, condition deteriorated, admitted in another hospital, Gangrene found and leg amputed upto thigh. District Forum allowed compensation.	7.5.1999	Appeal dismissed. Held, Negligence on the part of opposite party established. Allowed compensation Rs. 48,000 and cots Rs. 1,000.
192.	F.A. No. 818/97 I (2000) CPJ 288	Dr. Anumalla Satyanarayana v. K. Shankar	Andhra Pradesh, SCDRC, Hyderabad	Complainant suffering from pain in the right leg consulted opposite party kept under his own	10.5.1999	Appeal rejected. Held, doctor did not consulted any specialist and did not refer the complainant to any hospitals. Therefore, order of District

				diagnosis but no relief. In another hospital, leg got amputated because gangrene developed. District Forum allowed the compensation for Rs. 48,000 and cost Rs. 1000. Hence appeal was made.		Forum upheld and complainant is entitled to compensation.
193.	A. N. 542/95 I (2000) CPJ 433	Dr. Rameshwar P.D. Agrawal v. M.D. Abas Ansari	Bihar, SCDRC, Patna	Complainant got operated for removal of uterus. Hole occurred in urinary bladder while removing uterus then tube from urinary bladder was removed. District Forum allowed compensation of Rs. 53,685 and cost Rs. 1000. Hence appeal was made.	10.5.1999	Appeal allowed. Held, possibility of occurrence of V.V.F. (Vesico Vaginal Fistula) during such operation cannot be ruled out. Doctor exhibited expert skill in performing hysterectomy and was not guilty of negligence.

194.	A. N. 974/1997 II (1999) CPJ 633	Charan Singh v. Khosla Hospital & Anr.	Punjab, SCDRC, Chandigarh	Negligence in treatment and post-operative care of cataract operation, second operation performed. Eye sight lost.	11.5.1999	Appeal dismissed. Held, no evidence produced to prove that wrong medicines were prescribed. No negligence proved as operation was performed with reasonable care.
195.	A. No. 357/98 II (2000) CPJ 345	N.S. Sahota v. New Ruby Hospital & Ors.	Punjab, SCDRC, Chandigarh	Complainant alleged that his wife died because of deficiency in services provided by opposite party in not properly diagnosing the disease. She was suffering from diabetes with hypertension with bronchopneumonia. She was a heart patient also. District Forum dismissed the complaint Hence appeal was made.	13.5.1999	Appeal dismissed. Held, doctor tried his best to save the life of the patient. No direct expert evidence was produced to prove negligence of the doctor.

196.	OC No. 16/91 II (2000) CPJ 384	Smt. Bhanpal v. Dr. Prakash Padode & Ors.	Madhya Pradesh SCDRC, Bhopal	Patient admitted for operation of Hernia. Patient died. Alleged that heavy dose of anaesthesia given.	24.5.1999	Complaint allowed with costs Rs. 2000 and compensation Rs. 1,75,000. Held, doctor was guilty of negligence and deficiency in service. Further held that the complainant was not in a position to exactly state the factual aspects of whatever took place inside, thus duty was casted upon doctor to prove that no negligence took place inside the operation theatre.
197.	C. No. 30/0/95 III (1999) CPJ 609	Dilip Kumar Biswas v. Kothari Medical Centre	West Bengal, SCDRC, Calcutta	Complainant alleged negligence in operation resulting in haemorrhage during operation, with the result vision of both eyes lost.	26.5.1999	Complaint dismissed. Held, no negligence in operation proved as no connection between haemorrhage and vision lost was established.
198.	A.N. 881/1995 II (1999) CPJ 682	Smt. Raj Kuwar Bai & Anr. v.	Maharashtra, SCDRC, Mumbai	Proper treatment not given. Gangrene developed.	18.6.1999	Appeal dismissed. Held, Doctor adopted established practice of treatment. District

		Dr. R. R. Dhoot, Dhoot Hospital		Amputation of leg below knee. District Forum held no negligence. Hence appeal was made.		Forum order upheld as no negligence proved.
199.	A. N. 850/98 I (2000) CPJ 66	Dr. Janaki S. Kumar & Anr. v. Mrs. Sarafunnisa	Kerala, SCDRC, Thiruvananthapuram	Sterilisation was done without consent. District Forum allowed compensation of Rs. 2,75,000.	21.6.1999	Appeal dismissed. Held, person giving consent must be aware of risk involved. Patient under general anaesthesia neither can understand the risk involved nor could give the consent. Thus, it was not informed consent.
200.	C. No. C-202/93 III (1999) CPJ 167	Smt. Jaiwati Vs. Parivar Seva Sanstha & Anr.	Delhi, SCDRC, New Delhi	Sterilisation operation failed	22.6.1999	Complaint dismissed. Held any method of sterilisation has certain failure rate i.e. risk of failure is inherent in the procedure. Hence no negligence was found.
201.	A. N. 601 & 604/98 I (2000) CPJ 81	Dr. P. N. Bhaskaran & Anr. v. Mrs. Molly	Kerala, SCDRC, Thiruvanathapuram	Complainant underwent MTP for termination of pregnancy. Pregnancy	23.6.1999	Appeal allowed. Held, no deficiency found on the part of the doctor as it was the case of early pregnancy and the

		Robinson & Anr.		not got terminated. Patient got herself discharged and second surgery done in another hospital where MTP was conducted successfully. Alleged deficiency on the part of first doctor. District Forum allowed compensation Rs. 15,000 and cost Rs. 500 hence appeal was made.		chance of missing the product being there. D & C was a approved procedure in that case, but the complainant got herself discharged.
202.	C. No. 56/1996 III (1999) CPJ 75	Rekha V. Kamble & Ors. v. Dr. M. M. Aggarwal & Ans.	Maharashtra, SCDRC, Mumbai	Complainant alleged negligence in operation. Patient died. There was intestinal obstruction which caused retention of water and urine.	13.7.1999	Complaint dismissed. Held, death was due to cardiac arrest and measures was taken but failed to revive the patient.

203.	F.A. No. 44/99 I (2000) CPJ 340	Dr. N. Lalitha Krishna v. Mrs. Deepa Nair	Andhra Pradesh, SCDRC, Hyderabad	Complainant approached doctor for MTP which was conducted but foetus remained in tact and growing. Then second MTP done. District Forum allowed compensation of Rs. 10,500 plus costs Rs. 500.	14.7.1999	Appeal partly allowed. Held ,there was deficiency on the part of doctor. Compensation provided is Rs. 5000 plus refund of charges paid plus costs Rs. 500.
204.	O. C. No. 72/96 III (1999) CPJ 535	Biharilal Thavait v. Dr. Prakash Ladikar	Madhya Pradesh, SCDRC, Bhopal	Complainant operated upon for polio free of cost. Alleged that doctor cheated him by advising him for five year not to fold his leg with the result, he is not in a position now to fold his legs at all.	29.7.1999	Complaint dismissed. Held that operation was performed free of costs. Further the complaint was time-barred. The complaint was found to be frivolous/vexatious as doctor had done best with the best of his expertise and ability.
205.	A.N. 949/97 III (2000) CPJ 366	Dr. M.S.Khatambre v. Babu K. Kople	Maharashtra, SCDRC, Mumbai	Complainants 7 month old child got treatment and	2.9.1999	Appeal allowed. Held, doctor was not negligent in the treatment.

				expired. District Fourm allowed compensation of Rs. 5000. Hence appeal was made.		
206.	A. N. 868/95 III (1999) CPJ 546	Dr. R. K. Jain v. Sunil	Madhya Pradesh, SCDRC, Bhopal	Complainant's son got burnt, got treatment but son became invalid. District Forum allowed complaint. Hence appeal was made.	6.9.1999	Appeal allowed. Held complainant filed affidavit of one Dr. Agrawal, B.A.M.S. who is not competent to give expert evidence. Further nexus between treatment and virus leading to invalidness not proved. Complainant failed to prove negligence.
207.	C.C. No. 29/98 II (2000) CPJ 262	Jaswinder Singh & Ors. v. Dr. J. S. Saini & Anr.	Union Territory of CDRC, Chandigarh	Patient operated upon for eye deformity by births. But deformity ever increased.	6.10.1999	Complaint allowed with costs Rs. 5000 and compensation Rs. 2,00,000 as negligence is well established on the part of the doctor and PGI, Chandigarh.

208.	O.C. No. 75/96 I (2000) CPJ 129	Syed Zahid Ali v. Dr. Jai Prakash Paliwal	Madhya Pradesh, SCDRC, Bhopal	Complaint alleged negligence in operation. Non-removal of gauge from inside the body.	18.10.99	Complaint dismissed with costs Rs.·2000 under section 26. Held, Complaint found to be frivolous. Complainant filed no document in support of contention. Held, complaint was false.
209.	A.N. 447/97 I (2000) CPJ 361	Smt. Chandra v. Dr. Mahesh & Ors.	Tamil Nadu, SCDRC, Chennai	Complainant alleged that operation was performed in a hurried and hasty manner. Two operations were performed for removal of lump.	25.10.99	Appeal dismissed. Held, operation was performed only after clinical examination and according to standard medical practice. Further, no material evidence produced to prove gross negligence.
210.	A.N. 158/99 III (2000) CPJ 354	K.E. Rajesh v. The President, District Cooperative Hospital & Anr.	Kerala state, SCDRC, Thiruvananthapuram	Complainant undergone an operation in a co-operative hospital. Resulting in pain not relieved, had to undergo another operation. Complainant was a	1.11.1999	Complaint is maintainable. Referred to District Forum.

				manual labour. Alleged his daily earning was affected by negligence in operation. District Forum dismissed the complaint. Hence appeal was made.		
211.	C.No. 100/98 III (2000) CPJ 407	S.K. Sharma v. Dr. P.B. Desai	Maharashtra, SCDRC, Mumbai	Complainant and wife treated by doctor for breast cancer, wife expired.	20.12.99	Complaint dismissed. Held, there was no error of judgement. Doctor adopted the best and correct method.
212.	C.No. 12/97 II (2000) CPJ 439	Jaspal Singh & Anr. v. The Post Graduate Institute of Medical Education and Research, PGI Chandigarh	Union Territory CDRC, Chandigarh	Complaint's wife suffered burn injuries to the extent of 50% admitted to PGI. Patient's blood group was A+ but doctor transfused B+ group blood. As a result kidney damaged. patient died.	1.2.2000	Complaint allowed. Held there was mismatching of blood group and wrong trans-fusion. PGI Chandigarh was liable to pay compensation of Rs. 2,00,000.

213.	O.C. No. 56/96 II (2000) CPJ 463	S.A. Qureshi v. Padode Memorial Hospital & Research Centre	Madhya Pradesh, SCDRC, Bhopal	Patient undergone a knee joint operation, resulting in permanent disability. Hospital was silent to explain the cause of disability as they made plea of elimination of records.	2.2.2000	Complaint allowed with costs Rs. 550 and compensation Rs. 50,000. Held, plea of elimination of record approve to be an attempt to suppress certain facts.
214.	A. No. 970/99 II (2000) CPJ 293	Suraj Singh Vs. Dr. Manoj Kankaney	Uttar Pradesh, SCDRC, Lucknow	Patient got plastered in a fractured arm. Alleged negligence on the part of doctor as patient was not able to move his finger. District Forum dismissed the complaint with the costs Rs. 400. Hence appeal was made.	6.3.2000	Appeal dismissed. Held, no opinion of any doctor was filed. However, there was a certificate that complainant had broken the plaster. District Forum's order confirmed.

215.	O.C. No. 57/96 (II (2000) CPJ 441	Malkhan Singh v. Modern X-ray Sonography and Patho Centre & Anr.	Madhya Pradesh, SCDRC, Bhopal	Complainant alleged for wrong sonography report stating death of foetus on that the complainant got his wife aborted.	13.4.2000	Complaint dismissed without costs. Held, sonography report was not wrong. Hence, no deficiency in service proved.
216.	O. C. No. 18/95 II (2000) CPJ 502	Abdulla Modiwala & Sons v. G. D. Birla Memorial Health Centre & Ors.	Madhya Pradesh, SCDRC, Bhopal	Complainant's wife suffering with bleeding undergone a tubectomy operation. Died during operation.	24.4.2000	Complaint dismissed. Held, complainant failed to produce evidence, expert opinion as the burden of establishing negligence is on the complainant's.
217.	A.N. 145/98 II (2000) CPJ 566	Pushpabai v. Dr. S. Joseph	Madhya Pradesh, SCDRC, Bhopal	Complainant conceived after tubectomy operation. District Forum dismissed the complaint as she has made no payments. Hence appeal was made.	25.4.2000	Appeal dismissed. Held complainant was not a consumer under the Act as free services were provided. Further expert evidence was not produced to prove negligence and no method of tubal sterilisation is without failure.

218.	C. No. 28/95 II (2000) CPJ 220	Ashok Kumar Singh v. Dr. Mohan Thakur	Bihar, SCDRC, Patna	Complainant suffered multiple injury in leg. Treatment took very long, still fractured leg bone was not joined.	2.5.2000	Complaint dismissed. Held, no evidence was there to show that fractured bone took long to unite. At the time of examination, fractured bone got united.
219.	OP No. 67/2000 (I (2001) CPJ 68)	Dr. M. Dravidamani v. Dr. S. Paramasivam	Tamil Nadu, SCDRC, Chennai	Complainant a diabetic had a blister in his left leg. then his thumb of leg removed than a portion of his left leg removed.	16.6.2000	Complaint dismissed in Limine. Held, no prima facie document was there to reveal negligence. Thus, no use to issue notice to opposite party which would likely to harass the opposite party.
220.	A.N. 47/99 I (2001) CPJ 8	Amar Singh v. Francis Newton Hospital & Ors.	Punjab, SCDRC. Chandigarh	Complainant's father aged 89 years admitted to hospital for weakness of left side of body, died. District Forum dismissed the complaint Hence, appeal was made.	26.6.2000	Appeal dismissed with costs Rs. 5000. Held, no evidence produced. Whereas report of Board of Doctors and cancellation of FIR lodged by complainant strengthened the case of the doctor.

221.	A. No. 941/98 I (2001) CPJ 197	Avtar Singh Bhatora v. Dr. Swarn Parkash Garg	Punjab, SCDRC, Chandigarh	Doctor not qualified and authorised to practice in allopathic system of medicine, prescribed allopathic drug for mninimising chest pain. Pain aggravated.	10.7.2000	Appeal allowed, compensation granted Rs. 5000 . Held it is a prima facie case of negligence, doctor was not qualified for prescribing allopathic medicine.
222.	OP No. 127/2000 I (2001) CPJ 137	V. Chandrasekhar v. Malar Hospitals Ltd.	Tamil Nadu, SCDRC, Chennai	Complainant having severe chest pain underwent coronary angiogram and angioplasty. Not satisfied with the treatment, undergone bypass surgery. Alleged wrong diagnosis.	22.9.2000	Complaint rejected in lemine. Held, diagnosis is forming of opinion on examination of patient and opinion may vary from one medical expert to another. Thus, wrong diagnosis is not amount to deficiency in service.
223.	CC No. 74/95 I (2001) CPJ 42	Manish Agarwal v. Administrator. Kamla Nehru Memorial Hospital	Uttar Pradesh, SCDRC, Lucknow	Complainant alleged that on the discharge certificate male child was written but female child was handed over. DNA	1.11.2000	Complaint dismissed with cost Rs. 3000. Held, complainant had not conducted DNA test. Other paper clearly showed that female child was born.

				test required to be conducted in order to ascertain the dispute.		
224.	A.No. 214/99 I (2001) CPJ 478	Ashok Kumar v. Dr. Suresh Sharma	Punjab, SCDRC Chandigarh	Complainant met an accident and knee joint fractured, got operated. Lower portion not united with rest of the patella causing pain and restricted movements. Plaster was changed twice. District Forum dismissed the complaint Hence. Appeal was made.	18.12.00	Appeal dismissed. Held, no expert evidence produced to prove negligence. Treatment was not against prescribed norms under medical jurisprudence.
225.	CC No. 79/SC/92 I (2001) CPJ 495	Raj Kumar v. Dr. Ajay Gupta & Ors.	Uttar Pradesh, SCDRC, Lucknow	Complainant's wife taken for pathological examination. Alleged that wrong report was given. Patient suffering from cancer not diagnosed. Patient died.	5.1.2001	Complaint dismissed. Held, pathological Dept. had submitted their report. Doctor was radiologist. In ultrasound, the cancer if it is less than 2 cms, cannot be detected. Thus no negligence established.

cent) were decided in favour of the patients where negligence on the part of the doctor or the health institution was proved. In 146 cases (64.89 per cent) negligence on the part of doctor or health institution was not established. Six cases were remanded back to the District Forums for fresh consideration and 16 cases (7.1 per cent) did not fall under the purview of the Consumer Protection Act as these were related to free services provided. In one of the cases, while dismissing the appeal, it was upheld by the Bihar State Consumer Disputes Redressal Commission, Patna that as a matter of policy and principle where subject matter was subjudice before the ordinary court a concurrent adjudication should not be conducted under the CPA, 1986. Hence subject matter was subjudice before the High Court.

The Consumer Courts also do not entertain complaints involving fraud, coercion and compulsion.

It has been revealed that death was not the main ground for making complaints in 72 per cent of cases (162 out of 225). More than fifty per cent of the cases (53.78 per cent i.e., 121 out of 225) were related to treatment involving surgery rather than to non-surgical treatment.

Regarding fees charged by the doctors, it was upheld by the Haryana State Consumer Disputes Redressal Commission, Chandigarh that the doctor could fix his fees; there could be no yard stick, as it differed from doctor to doctor.

Further, in case of *T. Rama Rao vs. Vijaya Hospital and Anr.* the Tamil Nadu State Consumer Disputes Redressal Commission, Chennai made it clear that the hospital could not be held vicariously liable for the negligence of the doctor when the doctor was paying rent to the hospital for using the space.

3.6 Conclusion

The study indicates that there is a fairly comprehensive framework for the regulation of medical services in India. However, the Indian Medical Council Act does not contain any provision for providing compensation to aggrieved patients. The

Civil Courts involved costs, time and procedural formalities. The Consumer Protection Act, 1986, is compensation-oriented and enacted to provide speedy and inexpensive justice with minimum formalities.

From the review the major cases decided by the National Commission and various State Commission set up under the Consumer Protection Act, 1986, it can be concluded that the Consumer courts have conducted themselves judiciously and that they have taken both letter and spirit of the law into account.

Furthermore, with the landmark judgement of the Supreme Court in the *Indian Medical Association v. V.P. Shantha* delivered in 1995, the awareness and confidence of the patients in the grievance redressal system under the CPA has considerably increased. While it is not always that the verdict of the Consumer Courts have gone in favour of the patient, they have also dismissed a number of complaints where the complainants failed to prove negligence on the part of the doctor. In the case of frivolous and vexatious complainants the Consumer Courts have taken a serious view and penalised the complainant.

The main ground for filing complainants against doctors and health institution was not that of death; rather than other consequences (in 60.38 per cent of the cases decided by the National Commission and in 72.00 per cent of the cases decided by various State Commissions). Furthermore, complaints were largely related to the deficiency in surgical treatment at against non-surgical treatment (62.26 per cent of the cases decided by the National Commission and in 53.78 per cent of the cases decided by various State Commissions).

Notes

1. Tandon, M.P. and Rajesh Tandon (1984), The Indian Penal Code (Faridabad: Allahabad Law Agency), p.285.

2. Ibid.

3. Ibid.

4. Ibid.

5. As quoted in Jesani, Amar and Vimla, Nandkani (1993) Patients Rights : A Perspective. The Indian Journal of Social Work (Tata Institute of Social Science), April, pp. 167-171.

6. Ibid.

7. (1992), CPJ 302 (NC).

8. Act No. 68 of 1986; Government of India, Gazette of India. (Extra ordinary). Part II, Section 1, No.83, dated December 26, 1986: Act No. 68 of 1986.

9. Government of India, Gazette of India, 1993 (Extra ordinary) Part II Section 1, No.84 dated June 18, 1993.

10. Dr. C.S. Subramanaoam vs. Kumarasamy and Anr. 1994 (3) CPR 403.

11. Inserted vide Consumer Protection (Amendment) Act, 1993.

12. Modified vide Consumer Protection (Amendment) Act, 1993.

13. Punjab National Bank, Bombay vs. K.B. Shetty 1991 (2) CPR 633: 1991 (2) CPJ 639 NC.

14. Motibai Dalvi Hospital vs. M.I. Govilkar 1992(1) CPR 408; 1991(2) CPJ 684.

15. Mumbai Grahak Panchayat vs. Andhra Pradesh Scooters Ltd., 1991(1) CPR 603.

16. The New India Assurance Co. Ltd., vs. M/s Green Transport Co. II(1991) CPJ 1 (Delhi).

17. Upbhogata Sanrakshan Manch vs. M/s Windsor Foods Ltd., 1993(2) CPR 608.

18. Commissioner of Transport vs. Y.R. Grover 1994(1) CPJ 199 National Commission.

19. Gulf Trivandrum Air Fare Forum vs. The Chairman and Managing Director, Air India 1992(2) CPJ 507.

20. M/s Krishna Conductors Pvt. Ltd., vs. Andhra Bank 1992(1) CPJ 176 NC.

21. S.K. Abdul Sukur vs. State of Orissa and Ors. II(1991) CPJ 202 (NCDRC): M/s Special Machines vs. Punjab National Bank and Ors. I(1991) CPJ 78.

22. Punjab National Bank vs. K.B. Shetty II(1991) CPJ 639 NC.

23. Branch Manager LIC of India and Anr. vs. Smt. Zareena Sulaiman 1995(1) CPJ 4.

24. Ibid.

25. III. (1995) CPJ 1 SC.

26. Cosmopolitan Hospital & Anr. v. Vasantha, P. Nair, I (1992) CPJ 302 (NC).

27. K.B. Jayalaxmi vs. Govt. of Tamil Nadu and Ors. 1994(1) CPR 114.

28. Ibid.

29. M/s Spring Meadows Hospital & Anr. v. Harjot Ahluwalia, through K.S. Ahluwalia & Anr., III (1998) CPJ 1 SC.

30. Verma, D.P.S. The Consumer Protection Act : A New Challenge to the Marketing Manager a paper presented at the faculty seminar on Business Strategy in Regulated Environment, New Delhi, March, 1987.

31. Consumer Unity and Trust Society, Jaipur v. State of Rajasthan and Others (First Appeal No.2 of 1989, decided on 15.12.1989).

32. Inserted vide The Consumer Protection (Amendment) Act, 1993.

33. III (1995) CPJ 1 SC.

34. A.C. Modagi v. Cross Well Tailors and Another} (Revision Petition No.75 of 1990, decided on 9.8.1991).

35. Per Hilbery, J. in Collins v. Hertfordshire Country Council} 1947 KB 598 at Page 615 as quoted in Dharangadhra Chemical Works Ltd. v. State of Saurashtra and Others} {, AIR 1957 SC 264 at p.267.

36. 1910-1 KB 543 at pp.549-550.

37. A.C. Modagi vs. Cross Well Tailor and Anr. 1991(2) CPR 432; II (1991) CPJ 586 (NC); Kasturi Bhattacharjee vs. Sivaji Basu and Ors. I (1997) CPJ 575.

38. Ibid.

39. Smt. Rohini Pritam Kabadi vs. Dr. R.T. Kulkarni III (1996) CPJ 441.

40. Pavitar Singh and Ors. vs. State of Punjab and Anr. I (1994) CPJ 397: S.S. Kahlon and Anr. vs. Bawa Hospital and Ors. III (1994) CPJ 286.

41. The Additional Director, CGHS, Pune vs. Dr. R.L. Butani I (1996) CPJ 255 (NC).

42. Treasury Officer and Other Member Secretary, Pensioner Medical Fund and Ors. Vs. G.K. Joshi I (1996) CPJ 22.

43. 2000 (1) CCC 162 (NS).

44. The Consumer Protection Act, 1986, Chapter II.

45. Ibid., Chapter III.

46. Ibid., Section 4.

47. Ibid., Section 7.

48. The Consumer Protection Act, 1986, Section 4, read with Rule 3 of the Consumer Protection Rules, 1987.

49. Consumer Protection Rules, 1987, Rule 3(2).

50. The Consumer Protection Act, 1986, Section 5(1).

51. Ibid., Rule 4(5).

52. Ibid., Section 9(1).

53. Ibid., Section 7(2).

54. Ibid., Section 8. see also section 6.

55. The Consumer Protection Act, 1986, Section 10(1).

56. The Consumer Protection Act, 1986, Section 10(2).

57. The Consumer Protection Act, 1986, Section 9(b).

58. Ibid., Section 16(1) (a).

59. Ibid., Section 16(1) (b).

60. Ibid., Provision to Section 16(1).

61. Ibid., Section 16(2).

62. Common Cause v. Union of India (1989) 2 scale 541 and Common Cause v. Union of India(1993) scale 17.

63. Ashok Bhai R. Shah vs. Vijyaben 1993(1) CPR 347.

64. Jhunjunwala Bros. vs. Subbaramier (Alagiriswami J.) AIR 1968 Madras 194.

65. Consumer Education and Research Society vs. Skypak Couriers P. Ltd. 1991(2) CPR 462 p. 465: 1992(3) CPJ 111.

66. Sandeep Maini vs. Director, Meghalaya State Lottery 1992(1) CPJ 291.

67. Sanjeev Kumar vs. Rockland Leasing Ltd. 1993(2) CPR 186: Shimla Development Authority vs. Yash Pal Dass and Anr. 1992(3) CPJ 606.

68. M.P. Oxide Batteries (P) Ltd., vs. M.P. Electricity Board 1994(3) CPJ 41 NC.

69. Harbhajan Singh vs. Dayanand Medical College and Hospital and Ors. III (1996) CPJ 263.

70. P.P. Ismail vs. Kerala State Consumer Disputes Redressal Commission and Ors. II (1994) CPJ 449 (Kerala High Court).

71. The Consumer Protection Act, 1986, Section 13(4), read with Section 18 and 22 and Rule 10 of the Consumer Protection Rules, 1987.

72. The Consumer Protection Rules, 1987, Rule 10(1).

73. The Consumer Protection Act, 1986, Section 24.

74. The Hindustan Times, March 13, 1993.

75. The Hindustan Times, April 10, 1993.

76. For detail see : Singh, M.P. (1990), V.N. Shukla's Constitution of India (Lucknow : Eastern Book Co.) pp. 217, 440.

77. Tulasi Enterprises v. AP State Consumer Commission, AIR 1991 AP 326; Calcutta Metropolitan Development Authority v. Union of India, AIR 1993 Cal 4; Smt. N. Taneja v. Calcutta District Forums, AIR 1992 Cal.; For a critical analysis of relevant cases on this subject see : Singh, S.N. (1992) Jurisdiction issues before a Consumer Protection Forum Corporate Law Adviser (March) pp.96-101.

78. II (1994) CPJ 449 (Kerala High Court).

79. The Consumer Protection Act, 1986, Section 25.

80. 1991 (I) CPR 276.

81. Brij Mohan Kher vs. Dr. N.H. Banka and Anr. I (1995) CPJ 99 NC.

82. K. Jayaraman vs. The Poona Hospital and Research Centre and Ors. III (1993) CPJ 402 (NC).

83. III (1995) CPJ 1 SC.

Chapter 4

Patients' Perception of Medical Services in India

The objective of this chapter is to assess the perception of patient's about medical services provided by doctors and health institutions and the desirability of the CPA as a means of redressal against deficiency in medical services.

Having felt the need for an independent and systematic study of the patients' perception of services provided by doctors and health institutions, a survey of 540 patients of private and government health institutions was conducted with a view to determine the extent to which patients feel satisfied with the services provided to them by doctors and health institutions. Patients were selected keeping in mind that the sample represents five major specialities, viz., medicine, surgery, obstetrics and gynaecology, paediatrics and orthopaedics. Age, sex, education, occupation and income were the chief considerations which helped in selecting the respondents. The study covered patients who were receiving services in the out-patient departments (OPDs), those who were actually admitted in the health institutions, and those who had undergone some surgical operation. The survey was conducted in Delhi through personal interview, with the help of a direct, structured and non-disguised questionnaire. The profile of the patients is presented below:

4.1 Profile of the Sample: Patients

In order to have an insight about the patients' opinion about the medical services provided, it was decided to select the patients having different demographic characteristics. A profile of the patients on the basis of these characteristics is presented in Table 4.1.

The age-wise distribution of patient-respondents revealed that out of 540 patients, 126 (23.3 per cent) were up to 30 years of

Table 4.1: Profile of Patient-respondents

Demographic Characteristics	Patients Number	Patients Per cent
Distribution by Age:		
Up to 30 years	126	23.3
31 to 50 years	232	43.0
More than 50 years	182	33.7
Total	540	100.0
Distribution by Sex:		
Male	280	51.0
Female	260	48.1
Total	540	100.0
Distribution by Education:		
Illiterate	66	12.2
Up to Higher Secondary	164	30.4
Graduate	216	40,0
Post-graduate and Professionally qualified	94	17.4
Total	540	100.0
Distribution by Occupation:		
Government Service	96	17.8
Private Service	78	14.4
Business	76	14.1
Profession	42	7.8
Housewife	146	27.0
Retired employee	56	10.4
Others (Students and Farmers)	46	8.5
Total	540	100.0
Distribution by Income:		
Below Rs. 3,000	120	22.2
Rs. 3,000 - Rs. 10,000	266	49.3
More than Rs. 10,000	154	28.5
Total	540	100.0
Distribution by Type of Health Institution:		
Government Hospital	136	25.2
Private Hospitals	404	74.8
Total	540	100.0

age, 232 (43 percent) were in the age group of 31 years to 50 years, and 182 (33.7 per cent) were above 50 years of age.

Out of the total 540 patients, 280 (51.9 percent) were males and 260 (48.1 percent) were females.

Classified on the basis of education, 12.2 percent of the respondents were illiterate, 30.4 percent had qualification up to higher secondary, 40 percent were graduates and 17.4 percent were post-graduates and professionally qualified.

Occupation-wise, 17.8 percent of the patients were government servants, 14.4 percent were in private service, 14.1 percent had their own business, 7.8 percent were professionals, 27 percent were housewives, 10.4 percent were retired employees and 8.5 percent were in others categories, including students and farmers.

The distribution of patient-respondents on the basis of their monthly income were like this. Out of the 400 responding patients, 22.2 percent had their income below Rs. 3,000 per month, 49.3 percent respondents had income ranging from Rs. 3,000 to Rs. 10,000 per month, and 28.5 percent had more than Rs. 10,000 per month.

Since the services provided free of cost are excluded from the ambit of the CPA, and such services are, by and large, provided by government hospitals, the main concern was to study the opinion of the patients who got private medical services on payment basis. Therefore, approximately 75 percent of patients (404 out of 540) were those who were getting medical services from private doctors and health institutions both free as well as on payment basis. However, in order to have an insight into the perception of patients of government hospitals, approximately 25 percent of patients (136 out of 540) were also interviewed. These patients were receiving medical services from government hospitals both free as well as on payment basis.

A look at the profile of the patients in Table 4.1 reveals that the sample is representative enough in the sense that the respondents included patients of different age groups, income levels, occupations and education levels.

In order to assess the patients' perception about the services provided by doctors and health institutions, they were asked questions about the reasons for choosing a particular doctor or health institution, waiting time for doctors, behaviour of hospital personnel, quality of services provided to them at various levels including registration, nursing, doctors and investigations, information provided to patients, patients satisfaction with medical services received, and in the case of dissatisfaction, the actions taken by the patients, their expectations from the medical profession, the reasons for the patients bringing complaints, and their perception about the role of the CPA in patients' grievance redressal against deficiency in medical services.

In addition to the above questions, a few more questions were addressed to the patients who were admitted in the hospital and also to the patients who had undergone some surgical operation, with a view to gather their opinion about the services received by them during their stay in the hospital.

Out of the total of 540 patients, 260 patients (48.14 percent) were those who were admitted in the hospital during the time the survey was conducted. Out of these 260, 118 patients were those who had undergone some kind of surgery. The rest of the 280 patients (51.9 percent) were those who were receiving services in the out-patient departments (OPDs).

4.2 Patient's Perception Regarding Medical Services

An analysis of the responses of the patients is summarised in the following paragraphs.

4.2.1 Reasons for Patients' Choice of a Health Institution: In reply to the query whether they were already taking treatment for the present illness before coming to the health institution, when they were interviewed, 300 patients (55.6 percent) responded that they were already taking treatment. The reasons for which the patients stopped consulting their previous doctor or health institution are presented the Table 4.2. Out of the 300 patients, 23.30 percent were not satisfied. A very large number of patients

(76.7 percent) were referred to the hospital by the doctor they were consulting. It implies that a vast majority of patients go to the hospital, which their doctors prescribe.

The major reasons that emerged for patient's choice of a particular hospital were as follows: (1) faith and popularity of the doctor (44.4 percent), (2) referred by a doctor (38.1 percent), (3) convenience of location (33.7 percent), and (4) faith and popularity of the health institutions (31.1 percent).

Table 4.2: Reasons for Patients Discontinuing Consultations with the Doctor

Reasons	No. of patients	Percent
Not satisfied with service	70	23.3
Referred to such hospital	230	76.7
Total	**300**	**100.0**

The major reasons indicated by the patients for choosing a government hospital and a private hospital emerged out to be somewhat different. The first four major reasons for choosing the particular health institution by the patients of private and government hospitals are summarised in Table 4.3.

Table 4.3: Reasons for Patients' Choice of a Particular Health Institution: Government vs. Private

Major reason for choosing a government hospital	No. of patients (percent) N=136
Referred by a doctor	86 (63.2)
Free of cost	60 (44.1)
Faith and popularity of health institution	54 (39.7)
Specialist in this type of illness	40 (29.4)

Contd..

Major reason for choosing a private hospital	No. of patients (percent) N=404
Faith and popularity of doctor	234 (57.9)
Convenience of location	154 (38.1)
Referred by a doctor	120 (29.7)
Faith and popularity of health institution	(114 (28.2)

The top two reasons emerged out in case of patients of government hospitals were : (1) referred by a doctor and (2) free of cost. While in the case of patients of private hospitals' patients, (1) faith and popularity of doctor and (2) convenience of location, emerged out to be the top two reasons for choosing a particular private hospital.

4.2.2 Patients' Expectations from Medical Profession: In order to determine the patients' expectations from medical profession, patients were asked to rank their expectations in order of preference. A large majority of the patients (83 percent) expected 'immediate attention' which got the highest rank (1) from the patients.

Besides 'immediate attention', patients expected 'proper diagnosis' as their second preference. The third major concern of the patients, in addition to 'immediate attention' and 'proper diagnosis' was 'reasonable charges' on the one hand, and 'doctor's sympathetic behaviour' on the other hand.

In addition to these, another major concern of the patients was to get more information about illness and treatment to patients from the doctor.

Thus, patients expect that they should be fully informed about what is happening to them, what treatment they are getting, its side-effects and risks and how they can prolong their life, this implies that they desire complete information about their illness and treatment. Health institutions and doctors should understand the patients' need, and try their best to be more communicative with their patients, which would be in the best interest of both the parties.

4.2.3 Patients' Opinion about the Services Rendered at OPD: With regard to the time, the patients have to wait for being attended by the doctor in the out-patient departments (OPDs), it has been revealed that in the case of government hospitals, only a few patients (5.9 percent) had to wait for 16-30 minutes. No patient, however, reported less than 15 minutes waiting time and half of the patients (50 percent) had to wait for more than one hour for being attended by the doctor. Furthermore, while personally interviewing, they reported that they even had to wait for 2 to 3 hours for the doctor.

In the case of private health institutions, more than half of the patients (52 percent) reported that it took them up to 15 minutes to wait for the doctor. Quite a good number of patients (43 percent) reported that they waited for 16-30 minutes. Very few (2.5 percent) and almost a negligible number of patients (1 percent) reported to have waited for the doctor for 31 minutes to one hour and more than one hour, respectively. Thus, it appears that in government hospitals, the patients have to wait for the longer period as compared to those in the private health institutions.

From the responses of the patients regarding the efficiency of the staff at the registration counter it has been observed that a large majority of patients (70.6 percent) in government hospitals felt that the staff at the registration counter was inefficient and unconcerned, while an overwhelming majority of the patients of private hospitals (94 percent) were of the view that their staff was efficient and helpful.

As regards the average time spent by the doctors in examining the patients, out of the 540 patients, 536 patients responded. A substantial majority of patients (81.9 percent) reported that the doctor spent up to five minutes to examine them. Only a negligible number of patients (2.6 percent) reported that the doctor spent more than 10 minutes to examine them. There did not seem to be much difference in the responses of patients of private hospitals and government hospitals. The majority opinion in the case of both types of hospitals was that the doctors did not spend more than five minutes in examining each patient.

Regarding the display of necessary facilities an overwhelming majority of patients (93.3 percent) reported that the necessary facilities including X-ray, ECG and C-T scan etc. were displayed at the counter. There appeared to be not much difference in the responses of patients of private and government hospitals. A majority of patients, in each of the categories, reported that necessary information about such facilities was displayed at the counter.

The patients' response as to whether the necessary information about the cost involved was provided to them beforehand or not revealed that in the case of government hospitals not many patients (25 percent) reported that cost information was provided beforehand. However, more than half of the patients of private hospitals (59.4 percent) got the cost information beforehand.

In total, out of 540 patients, 274 (50.7 percent) reported that they got the cost information beforehand. However, still a good number of patients (49.3 percent) were those who did not get the cost information beforehand.

Thus, it can be implied that the doctors and the health institutions are lacking in providing cost information to patients beforehand.

4.2.4 Patients' Satisfaction with the Quality of Medical Services: The patients's satisfaction about the quality of services provided by the health institutions was measured on a five point scale ranging from most satisfactory to most dissatisfactory, with regard to various indicators of services including reception, administration, cleanliness, nursing staff, doctors, investigations, supply of written records, and medical store.

Responses were collected and mean scores were found out. Score 1 was given to the most satisfactory and 5 to the most dissatisfactory, this implies that lesser the mean score, better would be the satisfaction level, f-test for analysis of variance was applied among various groups of demographic characteristics including age, sex, education, income and the type of health institutions (government and private), in order to determine whether there was a significant difference in their satisfaction level regarding quality of medical service provided. The results are presented in Table 4.4.

Table 4.4: Patients' Satisfaction with Quality of Medical Services

Demographic variables	Number of Patients	Mean (X)	Standard Deviation (S.D.)	F-ratio	F probability
Age:					
Up to 30 years	126	19.60	3.66		
31-50 years	232	19.87	3.61	0.6	0.5
More than 50 years	182	19.67	3.69	(Not significant)	
Total	540	19.67	3.69		
Educational Qualification:					
Illiterate	66	19.54	2.85		
Upto Higher Secondary	164	19.93	3.76	0.57	0.63
Graduate	216	19.67	3.74	(Not significant)	
Post-graduate and Professionally qualified	94	19.32	3.99		
Total	540	19.67	3.69		
Sex:					
Male	280	20.01	3.8	4.97	0.02
Female	260	10.30	3.50	(Significant at 2%)	
Total	540	19.67	3.69		
Income					
Upto Rs. 3,000	120	19.58	2.58		
Rs.3000-Rs.10,000	266	19.75	2.92	0.14	0.8
More than Rs.10000	154	19.60	4.01	(Not significant)	
Total	540	19.67	3.69		
Type of Health Institution					
Govt. Hospitals	136	22.31	4.15	111.50	0.00
Private hospitals	404	18.79	3.06	(Highly significant)	
Total	540	19.67	3.69		

Following observations can be made from the Table:

1. The satisfaction level did not differ significantly among

patients having various age groups. However, as compared to younger patients, patients above 50 years of age appeared to be more satisfied with the quality of medical services provided.

2. The patients satisfaction about the quality of services provided among patients having various educational levels did not differ significantly. However, post-graduate and professionally qualified patients seemed to be more satisfied in comparison to other patients.

3. There were significant differences in the opinion of male and female patients regarding the quality of medical services provided by health institutions. Female patients appeared to be more satisfied with the services, in comparison to male patients.

4. A highly significant difference was found in the satisfaction level of the patients of private and government health institutions. Patients of the private health institutions appeared to be much more satisfied in comparison to the patients of government hospitals.

4.2.5 Perception as to Behaviour of Staff of Health Institution: Patients' opinion about behaviour of staff, viz., polite, helpful and prompt is presented in Table 4.5. Patient's opinion as sought on a four-point scale (score 1 was given to 'always', 2 to 'generally', 3 to 'rarely' and 4 to 'never', which implies that lesser mean indicates greater satisfaction).

Mean scores were calculated for each sub-group of age, educational qualification, sex and type of health institution (government and private). f-test has been applied to determine whether there was significant difference in their opinion about behaviour of staff of health institution. Following observations are made from Table 4.5.

1. The patients' opinion did not differ significantly among various age groups as far as behaviour of the staff was concerned. however, as compared to other patients, patients below 30 years of age appeared to be more satisfied.

2. There was a significant difference in the opinion of patients having various educational qualifications as far as the

behaviour of staff was concerned. While illiterate patients appeared to be more satisfied with the behaviour of staff, graduate patients seemed to be less satisfied in comparison to the other patients.

Table 4.5: Perception as to Behaviour of Staff of Health Institution

Demographic variables	Number of Patients	Mean (X)	Standard Deviation (S.D.)	F-ratio	F probability
Age:					
Upto 30 years	126	23.71	5.68		
31-50 years	232	24.47	5.33	1.16	0.31
More than 50 years	182	23.78	5.41	(Not significant)	
Total	540	24.06	5.44		
Educational Qualification:					
Illiterate	66	23.21	5.40		
Upto Higher Secondary	164	23.52	5.71	3.24	0.02
Graduate	216	24.94	5.24	(Significant at 2%)	
Post-graduate and Professionally qualified	94	23.57	5.24		
Total	540	24.06	5.44		
Sex:					
Male	280	24.31	5.57	1.23	0.20
Female	260	23.79	5.30	(Not significant)	
Total	540	24.06	5.44		
Income					
Upto Rs. 3,000	120	24.17	5.34		
Rs.3000-Rs.10,000	266	24.22	5.75	0.47	0.61
More than Rs.10000	154	24.06	5.44	(Not significant)	
Total	540	19.67	3.69		
Type of Health Institution					
Govt. Hospitals	136	28.85	4.98	189.75	0.00
Private hospitals	404	22.45	4.58	(Highly significant)	
Total	540	24.06	5.44		

3. The difference in the opinion of male and female patients was not found to be significant. However, female patients appeared to be more satisfied in comparison to male patients.

4. There was a highly significant difference in the opinion of patients of government and private health institutions. The patients of the private hospitals seemed to be more satisfied in comparison to patients of government health institutions, as far as the behaviour of the staff was concerned.

4.2.6 Information about Illness and Treatment Provided by Doctors

Patients' opinions about information about their illness, options available for treatment, possible side-effects and complications, time required for recovery, causes of illness, treatment given, unforeseen consequences and risks involved and future lifestyle expected, are analysed according to the patients' educational qualifications, in order to determine whether there is any difference on the part of doctor in so far as they provide information to the patients having differing educational qualifications.

As shown in Table 4.6, a large majority of patients in all the four educational categories, viz., illiterate (97 percent), up to higher secondary (96.3 per cent), graduate (98.1 per cent) and post-graduate and professionally qualified (97.9 percent) reported that doctor provided them information regarding their illness. However, regarding the other aspects of information, it is evident from the Table that doctors were not providing adequate information: options available (8.1 percent), possible side-effects (15.9 percent), time required for recovery (8.9 percent), causes of illness (3.3 percent), treatment given (5.9 percent), unforeseen consequences and risks involved (3.3 percent) and future lifestyle to be adopted (2.2 percent).

Thus, there is no significant difference in the attitude of doctors to patients having different educational background so far as the provision of information about the illness and treatment is concerned.

Further, there seems to be a communication gap between the doctors and the patients. It appears that doctors consider patients as laymen and domestic not provide adequate information to patients. This gap needs to be bridged and doctors should provide adequate relevant information to patients about their treatment.

Table 4.6: Information about Illness and Treatment Provided by Doctors

Information About	No. of Patients (percent)				
	Illiterate	Upto Higher Secondary	Graduate	Post-graduate and Professionally qualified	Total
	N=66	N=164	N=216	N=94	N=540
Illness	64 (97)	158 (96.3)	212 (98.1)	92 (97.9)	526 (97.4)
Options available	6 (9.18)	28 (17.1)	6 (2.0)	4 (4.3)	44 (8.1)
Possible side effects	12 (18.2)	26 (15.9)	30 (13.9)	18 (19.1)	86 (15.9)
Time required for recovery	8 (12.1)	24 (14.6)	10 (4.6)	6 (6.4)	48 (8.9)
Causes of illness	0 (0)	8 (4.9)	6 (2.8)	4 (4.3)	18 (3.3)
Treatment given	2 (3)	10 (6.1)	16 (7.4)	4 (4.3)	32 (5.9)
Unforeseen consequences and risks involved	2 (3)	4 (2.4)	8 (3.7)	4 (4.3)	18 (3.3)
Future life style to be adopted	0 (0)	2 (1.2)	4 (1.9)	6 (6.4)	12 (2.2)

4.2.7 Perception as to the Necessity of Information Regarding Treatment

As shown in Table 4.7, a whopping majority of patients (97.4 percent) felt the necessity of asking the appropriate line of treatment and its unforeseen consequences and an overwhelming majority of patients (95.9 percent) actually asked the doctor regarding the appropriate line of treatment.

Table 4.7: Perception as to the Necessity of Information regarding Treatment

Particulars	No. of Patients (percent)				
	Illiterate	Upto higher secondary	Graduate	Post-graduate and professionally qualified	Total
	N=66	N=164	N=216	N=94	N=540
Patients feel the necessity of asking appropriate line of treatment	60 (90.9)	162 (98.8)	212 (98.1)	92 (97.9)	526 (97.4)
Actually asked about the appropriate line of treatment	56 (84.8)	156 (95.1)	212 (98.1)	94 (100.0)	518 (95.9)

When this aspect is analysed according to the education level of the patients, there does not seem to be much difference in the categories, up to higher secondary (98.8 percent), graduate (98.1 percent), and post-graduate and professionally qualified (98 percent). But in the case of illiterate patients, such number is a little less (91 percent) which implies that in comparison to other three categories, illiterate patients seem to feel somewhat less the need to ask the doctors about the line of treatment.

Similarly, in the case of actually asking the doctor, the percentage of patients who had actually asked the doctor was found to be increasing with the increase in their education level: illiterates (84.8 percent), up to higher secondary (95.1 percent), graduates (98.1 percent) and post-graduate and professionally qualified patients, (100 percent). Thus, educational qualifications do make some difference in the patients in getting the desired information from the doctors.

4.2.8 Patients' Satisfaction over Doctor's Response to Queries

Patients' satisfaction over the doctor's response towards their queries is shown in Table 4.8. Of all the patients who actually queried the doctors, only 39.4 percent were satisfied with the doctors' response towards their queries regarding treatment. However, majority of the patients (61 percent) were not satisfied with the doctors' response towards their queries. Moreover, as the education level of patients rises, they seem to be more and more dissatisfied with the doctors' response. A large majority of the illiterate category of patients (71.4 percent) seem to be satisfied, while not many (29.8 percent) of post-graduate and professionally qualified patients were satisfied. The satisfied patients having qualifications up to higher secondary and graduation were 48.7 percent and 28.3 percent respectively.

Table 4.8: Patient's Satisfaction over Doctor's Response to Queries

Particulars	No. of Patients (percent)				
	Illiterate	Upto higher secondary	Graduate	Post-graduate and professionally qualified	Total
	N=56	N=156	N=212	N=94	N=518
Satisfied with the doctors' response to their queries	40 (71.42)	76 (48.72)	60 (28.30)	28 (29.79)	204 (39.38)
Dissatisfied with the doctors' response to their queries	16 (28.57)	80 (51.28)	152 (71.70)	66 (70.21)	314 (60.62)

The level of satisfaction was measured on a four-point scale ranging from 'highly satisfied' to 'highly dissatisfied'. As the response in 'highly satisfied' was negligible and in 'highly dissatisfied' was none, these categories were combined with the nearest categories on the scale. As a result of this merger two categories, namely, 'satisfied' and 'dissatisfied' emerged and are shown in the Table 4.8.

4.2.9 Patients' Awareness about Grievance Redressal Under CPA

The patients' awareness about getting redressal of grievances against deficiency in medical services under the CPA is shown in Table 4.9. It is evident from the Table that not many patients (20.4 percent) were aware about the Consumer Protection Act, 1986, while, a large majority of the patients (80 percent) were still unaware.

Table 4.9: Awareness of Patients about CPA

Particulars	No. of Patients (percent)				
	Illiterate	Upto higher secondary	Graduate	Post-graduate and professionally qualified	Total
	N=66	N=164	N=216	N=94	N=540
Aware about the CPA	Nil	18 (11.0)	38 (17.60)	54 (57.40)	110 (20.4)
Not aware about the CPA	66 (100)	146 (89.0)	178 (82.40)	40 (42.6)	430 (79.6)

Analysing this aspect on he basis of educational qualification of patients, Table 4.9 shows that none of the illiterate patients was aware about the CPA. Only a handful to patients (11 percent) having qualification up to higher secondary, a few graduate patients (17.6 percent) and more than half of the post-graduate and professionally qualified patients (57.4 percent) were aware of the CPA. Thus, as the educational level increased, the percentage of patients who were aware about the CPA went up, but still, there was a wide gap in the awareness level of the patients about the CPA. Thus, there is a need to create awareness about the CPA in the public.

4.2.10 Patients' Overall Satisfaction with Medical Services

After getting the responses of patients with respect to various aspects of services provided by doctors and health institutions, a general question was asked about the satisfaction of patients with the services provided by health institutions, and the responses have been presented in Table 4.10.

Table 4.10: Patients' Overall Satisfaction with Medical Services

On the Basis of Education					
Particulars	No. of Patients (percent)				
	Illiterate	Upto higher secondary	Graduate	Post-graduate and professionally qualified	Total
	N=66	N=164	N=216	N=94	N=540
Satisfied	52 (78.8)	128 (78)	156 (72)	76 (81)	412 (76.3)
Dissatisfied	14 (21.2)	36 (22)	60 (28)	18 (19)	128 (23.7)

On the Basis of Nature of Health Institution:			
Particulars	No. of Patients (percent)		
	Government Hospitals N=136	Private Hospitals N=404	Total N=540
Satisfied	52 (38.3)	360 (89)	412 (76.3)
Dissatisfied	84 (61.7)	44 (11)	128 (23.7)

Though the patients expressed dissatisfaction on individual parameters of measuring levels of satisfaction in the previous analysis, it seemed surprising that a large majority of the patients (76.3 percent) reported satisfaction with medical services, in general. Only a few patients (23.7 percent) had reported dissatisfaction.

From the Table, it can be observed that on the basis of educational qualification, there does not seem to be much difference in the satisfaction level of patients.

Patients' satisfaction of government and private health institution is also presented in Table 4.10. It is evident from the Table that a large majority of patients (89 percent) of private hospitals reported satisfaction with the medical services, while a considerable majority of patients (61.7 percent) of the government hospitals expressed dissatisfaction with the medical services they received.

4.2.11 Action Taken by Dissatisfied Patients: The opinion of the dissatisfied patients about the action taken by them is presented in Table 4.11.

4.2.11.1 Patients Dissatisfied and Suffering Specific Damages: As shown in Table 4.11, out of 128 patients who were dissatisfied, 28 patients (21.9 percent) had suffered specific damages during the treatment. Two patients did not give any response.

4.2.11.2 Aggrieved Patients Needing Compensation: The number of patients who wanted to get compensation out of those who had suffered specific damages is shown in Table 4.11. An overwhelming majority of patients (92.9 percent) who had suffered specific damages responded that they would like to get compensation. As for the illiterate category, none of the patients reported suffering any specific damage, hence, for this category, responses for this aspect could not be collected. For the other three educational categories of patients, having qualification up to higher secondary (100 percent), graduation (87.5 percent) and post-graduation and professional qualification (100 percent) responded that they would like to get compensation.

4.2.11.3 Action taken by Patients Suffering Damages: The dissatisfaction expressed by the patients in the form of complaints should cause deep concern to the hospitals authorities because in service organisations like hospitals, patients' satisfaction is the major contributing factor for optimising operational efficiency.

Just to have an idea bout how many dissatisfied patients on an average make complaints, a question was asked, and responses collected in this respect are shown in Table 4.11.

Table 4.11: Action Taken by Dissatisfied Patients

Particulars	No. of Patients (percent)				
	Illiterate	Upto higher secondary	Graduate	Post-graduate and professionally qualified	Total
	N=14	N=36	N=60	N=18	N=128
Patients who were dissatisfied and suffered specified damages during treatment					
Yes	--	6 (16.7)	16 (26.7)	6 (33.3)	28 (21.(9)
No	14 (100)	30 (83.3)	42 (70)	12 (66.7)	98 (76.6)
No response	--	--	2 (3.3)	--	2 (1.5)
Patients who had suffered specific damages and wanted to get compensation:					
	N=0	N=6	N=16	N=6	N=28
Yes	--	6 (100)	14 (87.5)	6 (100)	26 (92.9)
No	--	0 (0)	2 (12.5)	0 (0)	2 (7.1)
Action taken by patients who had suffered specific damages:					
Action taken	N=0	N=6	N=16	N=6	N=28
Nothing	--	--	--	--	--
Complained to hospital authority	--	6 (100)	14 (87.5)	6 (100)	26 (92.9)
Complained to referring doctor	--	--	2 (12.5)	--	2 (7.1)

It is evident from the Table that an overwhelming majority of the patients (92.9 percent) made complaints to the hospital authority. While only two out of 28 patients (12.5 percent) made complaints to their doctor. However, there does not seem to be much difference in the attitude of patients in making complaints on the basis of their educational qualification.

4.2.11.4 Patients' Satisfaction with Remedial Measures: As shown in Table 4.12, all the patients who had made complaints were dissatisfied with the remedial measures. Patients reported that it was very difficult to reach the top authorities, and even after making complaints to the higher authorities, no prompt action was taken. Besides, there was no clear-cut procedure to informs the patients of the action taken by the top authorities on their complaints.

Table 4.12: Patients' Satisfaction with Remedial Measures

Particulars	No. of Patients (percent)				
	Illiterate	Upto higher secondary	Graduate	Post-graduate and professionally qualified	Total
	N=0	N=6	N=16	N=6	N=28
Patients satisfaction with the remedial measures, who had taken any action for their dissatisfaction:					
Satisfied with remedial action	Nil	Nil	Nil	Nil	Nil
Dissatisfied with remedial action	Nil	6 (100)	16 (100)	6 (100)	28 (100)

4.2.11.5 Action Proposed by Patients Dissatisfied with Remedial Measures: The response of the dissatisfied patients regarding the action taken by them is presented in Table 4.13. A substantial majority of the patients (85.7 percent) expressed that they would like to take legal remedy. Only four out of 28 dissatisfied patients reported that they could approach voluntary organisations or report to some media.

Further, the Table indicates that as the education level of

patients rises, more and more of them like to go in for legal remedy up to higher secondary (66.7 percent), graduate (87.5 percent) and post-graduate and professionally qualified (100 percent).

Of all the patients, who wanted to take legal remedy, a considerable majority of the patients (75 percent) opined that they would like to take legal remedy under the forums under the CPA. None of the patients wanted to approach the Medical Councils. Patients expressed that the Medical Councils are mainly dominated by doctors and they were not sure of getting redressal from them. Moreover, Medical Council of India cannot provide compensation which majority of patients wanted to get. This is shown by the previous analysis of responses of patients (Table 4.11). Merely 8.3 percent of patients expressed their desire to approach the Medical Associations and the same percentage of patients desired to approach the Civil Courts for getting redressal of their grievances. 8.3 percent of patients did not give any response to this aspect.

Further, it is evident from the Table that a considerable majority of the patients (66.7 percent) favoured the CPA because of its speedy nature in comparison to the Civil Courts. Another 22.2 percent of patients were in favour of the CPA as it had minimum procedural formalities to be followed. Further, 11.1 percent of the patients expressed that they wanted to get redressal of their grievance under the CPA for the reason that it was inexpensive.

Therefore, it appears that people are expecting the CPA to be speedier than any other forum. According to Justice V.B. Eradi, past president of the National Commission, it takes presently, on an average, one or two years to get the redressal, as against 90 days period prescribed by the Act. But still, one or two years time period is much less in comparison to the Civil Courts in which average time period is 8 to 10 years [1]. Thus, the government should take steps to increase the efficiency and speed of the CPA so that it is able to meet the 90 days redressal time specified in it.

Table 4.13: Action proposed by Patients Dissatisfied with Remedial Measures

Particulars	No. of Patients (percent)				
	Illiterate	Upto higher secondary	Graduate	Post-graduate and professionally qualified	Total
	N=0	N=6	N=16	N=6	N=28
Patients who were dissatisfied with remedial measures taken by health institution to their complaint; action proposed by them:					
Wanted to take legal remedy	--	4 (66.7)	14 (87.5)	6 (100)	24 (85.7)
Others	--	2 (33.3)	2 (12.5)	0 (0)	4 (14.3)
Patients wanted to take legal remedy under:	N=0	N=4	N=14	N=6	N=24
Medical Councils	--	0	0	0	0
Medical Associations	--	0	2 (14.3)	0	2 (8.3)
Civil Courts	--	0	2 (14.3)	0	2 (8.3)
Forums under the CPA,1986	--	4 (100)	8 (57.1)	6 (100)	18 (75.0)
Non-response	--	0	2 (14.3)	0	2 (8.3)
Patients wanted to take legal remedy under the CPA as it is:					
	N=0	N=4	N=8	N=6	N=18
Speedy	--	2 (50)	6 (75)	4 (66.7)	12 (66.7)
Inexpensive	--	0	2 (25)	0	2 (11.1)
With minimum formalities	--	2 (50)	0	2 (33.3)	4 (22.2)

4.2.12 Perceived Injustice to Patients by Doctors

A whopping majority of patients (97 percent) were of the opinion that some doctors were not doing justice to the patients while performing their duties.

There does not seem to be any difference in the opinion of patients availing services of government hospitals and private hospitals, regarding this aspect. An overwhelming majority of patients (97 percent) in both the government as well as the private hospitals were of the view that some doctors were not doing justice in performance of their duties.

When patients were asked to give the possible reasons for such injustice, a whopping majority of patients (98 percent) expressed commercialisation as the major reason. Another major reason according to a large majority of patients (79.4 percent) was that the doctors did not feel the need to provide the necessary information to the patients about their illness.

The patients' opinion clearly revealed that some doctors are not doing justice to their duties because of their money-mindedness and not realising the importance of providing information to the patients about their illness and treatment. The patients expressed that doctors considered them laymen who could not understand their illness. The doctors did not think it necessary to provide the patients, the information desired by them. Thus, the doctors do not provide the adequate information to the patients about their illness and treatment. In the process, the patients are not able to understand how they have to take the treatment, what its side-effects and risks are and what life style they have to follow.

Analysing this aspect from the point of view of patients of government and private health institutions, it has been found that in addition to commercialisation (97 percent) and doctors' not feeling the necessity of providing information to patients (87.9 percent), other major reasons for government doctors not doing justice to the patients include : overburdened with work (84.8 percent) and lack of proper facilities (80.3 percent). However, in the case of the private health institutions, the major two reasons that emerged were as follows: Commercialisation (99.5 percent) and doctors' not feeling necessity of providing information to patients (76.5 percent). The percentage of the patients expressing that doctors were overburdened with work (5.1 percent) and there was lack of proper facilities (4.1 percent) were only negligible in the case of private hospitals.

4.2.13 Perception Regarding Doctors' Professional Accountability

More than half of the patients (53 percent) opined that doctors did not feel accountable to any authority for their professional conduct.

An open-ended question was asked to the patients as to which authority doctors are accountable. Examining the responses of the patients, it can be concluded that a majority of patients felt doctors are accountable either to the doctors' body, the hospital authority or to the Civil Courts.

The patients who opined that doctors did not feel accountable said that doctors should be accountable to general public through some law or to the CPA.

4.2.14 Patients' Grievances against Doctors and Health Institutions

The opinion of the patients about the common causes of their dissatisfaction in bringing a complaint against a doctor or health institution are presented in Table 4.14.

It is evident from the Table that the most important factor that triggers the complaining behaviour of patients is the improper and unsympathetic behaviour of doctors and hospital staff (95 percent and 97 percent respectively). As regards the reasons related to medical components, a substantially large majority of patients were of the opinion that wrong diagnosis (94.4 percent), lack of investigative facilities (88.9 percent) and negligence in informing the potential risks, side-effects of drugs and tests (86.2 percent) and unnecessary investigations (85.6 percent) were the main causes of patients' dissatisfaction.

Table 4.14: Major Grievances against Doctors and Health Institutions

Reasons for Patients' Dissatisfaction	Patients	
	Number	Percent
Non-availability of doctors when required	132	24.4
Non-availability or inadequacy of other para-medical services	444	82.2
Wrong diagnosis	510	94.4
Unnecessary Investigation	462	85.6
Over prescription	332	61.5
Lack of Investigation facilities	480	88.9
Failure to advise hospitalisation when indicated by patients' condition	264	48.9
Negligence in informing patients of potential risks and side-effects of drugs and tests	466	86.3
Failure to obtain informed consent for procedures with inherent risks	42	7.8
Improper behaviour of the doctor	514	95.2
Improper behaviour of staff	528	97.8
Lack of cleanliness in the premises	476	88.1
Over-charging	434	80.4
Patient instigated by other persons	16	1.1
For blackmailing	0	0.0
Patients' inability to judge doctor's expert opinion in terms of fees charged	84	15.6

Among the other reasons, a substantial majority of patients (80.4 percent) felt that overcharging was the major reason for their dissatisfaction with doctors and health institutions.

During the interviews the patients expressed the opinion that the charges were not commensurate with services provided by health institutions. They added that health institutions had become business houses, highly motivated only by commercial interests. Further, they also complained of inadequate para-medical services, (82.2 percent) and lack of cleanliness in the premises (88.1 percent).

4.2.15 Perception Regarding CPA's Role for Grievance Redressal

The opinion of the patients regarding the CPA to be helpful in getting the redressal of their grievances and in checking deficiency in medical services is presented in Table 4.15. An overwhelming majority of patients (98.9 percent) opined that applicability of the CPA would be helpful in getting redressal of their grievances and in checking deficiency in medical services. They felt that the procedure employed in the CPA was less time-consuming, inexpensive and involved minimum formalities in comparison to the Civil Courts. Further they expressed that the Medical Council of India was mainly dominated by doctors and could not provide compensation to aggrieved patients. Thus, they found the Consumer Protection Act, 1986, to be beneficial to patients in getting the redressal of their grievances.

Table 4.15: Perception regarding CPA's Role for Grievances Redressal

Particulars	Patients	
	Number	Percent
Applicability of CPA to medical services would be helpful in getting redressal of patients grievances and in checking deficiency in medical services?		
Yes	534	98.9
No	6	1.1
Total	540	100

4.2.16 Indoor Patients' Perception: Additional Aspects

The patients who were admitted to the hospitals were asked some additional questions in order to ascertain their opinion regarding their stay in the hospital. Out of the 540 patients interviewed, 260 patients were those who were admitted to the hospitals.

Waiting Period for Admission: A considerable majority of the patients (75 percent) reported average waiting time to be reasonable. however, there seemed to be a contrast in the opinion of the patients of government and private hospitals regarding this aspect. In the government hospitals, an overwhelming majority of the patients (92 percent) reported average waiting time to be unduly long, while in the case of private hospitals an overwhelming majority of the patients (91.5 percent) reported average waiting time to be reasonable. Therefore, in comparison to government hospitals, private hospitals are far more efficient in this regard.

Display of Rates of Charges for Medical Services: A considerable majority of the patients (75 percent) reported that the charges were displayed at the appropriate place. A very large majority (82 percent) of the patients of private hospitals reported that the charges were displayed at the appropriate place. However, in the case of government hospitals, less than half of the patients (44 percent) reported that the charges were displayed at the appropriate place.

Patients' Average Waiting Time in the Ward: In order to know the patients' waiting time between the arrival of the patients in the ward and their attendance by a nurse, Junior doctor and Senior Doctor, three time intervals have been developed, i.e. less than 10 minutes, 10-30 minutes and more than 30 minutes. The 10-30 minutes interval was considered to be the normal waiting time. The first time interval was considered to be efficient and the third one most inefficient.

More than half of the patients (55 percent) reported that nurses arrived in less than 10 minutes after their arrival in the ward. But, when the government hospitals are compared with the private hospitals in this respect, it was merely 8 percent of patients in government hospitals who reported their attendance by nurses in less than 10 minutes, while majority of patients (66 percent) responded to this time interval in the private hospitals.

A good number of patients (32 percent) of the government hospitals and only negligible number of patients (3 percent) of the private hospitals reported arrival of nurse even after half an hour. Therefore, again efficiency of the private hospitals is shown in comparison to the government hospitals.

Arrival of Junior Doctor: In the case of attendance of patients by a junior doctor, more than a few patients (31 percent) reported that junior doctor arrived in less than 10 minutes, while the figures for other two intervals were 38 percent and 31 percent respectively. In this aspect also, there seems to be a contrast difference in terms of the government and the private hospitals. While none of the patients of the government hospitals reported arrival of a junior doctor in less than 10 minutes, quite a good number of patients (38 percent) of private hospitals reported this time interval. A large majority of the patients (72 percent) of the government hospitals reported a junior doctor's arrival after half an hour. however, not many (22 percent) of the patients of the private hospitals reported this time interval.

Arrival of Senior Doctor: None of the patients of the government hospitals reported that a senior doctor came in less than 10 minutes, after his arrival in the ward. However, 17.6 percent of patients of the private hospitals reported that a senior doctor came within 10 minutes. A negligible number of patients (4 percent) of the government hospitals and quite a good number of patients (34 percent) of the private hospitals reported that the senior doctor came between 10-30 minutes. A vast majority of patients (96 percent) of the government hospitals reported that a senior doctor arrived after 30 minutes, while less than half of the patients (47.6 percent) of the private hospitals reported this time interval. Thus, on this account also, private hospitals proved to be comparatively more efficient than government hospitals.

4.2.17 Perception of Patients Having Undergone Surgery: Additional Aspects

In order to know the experiences of patients who have undergone surgery, some additional questions were asked from them.

Out of 260 patients who were admitted, 118 patients were those who had undergone some kind of surgery. Patients' opinion regarding the information about the operation to be done, line of treatment, risks involved, cost of operation and the care provided during operation and post-operative care was sought and analysed from the point of view of the patients of the government and private hospitals in order to determine the differences in their opinion.

Provision of Information regarding Operation to be Done: All the patients who had undergone surgery reported that the doctor provided the information regarding operation to be done. however, when patients were asked whether the doctor explained about patients' condition, line of treatment, operation to be done, and risks involved before taking their consent for operation, the response was in the positive from less than fifty percent (42.4 percent) patients only. The position was worse in the case of government hospitals where only a negligible number of patients (7 percent) reported that doctor explained to them the nature of operation to be done before taking their consent. however, in the private hospitals more than half of the patients (53 percent) gave this viewpoint. Thus, it implies that doctors are not providing adequate information to patients even before taking their consent.

Provision of Information about Cost Involved in Operation: Regarding the information about cost involved, a large majority of patients (84.7 percent) reported that they had inquired about the probable cost of operation. While in the government hospitals, more than half of patients (57 percent) reported that they had inquired about the cost involved in the operation, in the private hospitals, a vast majority of patients (93 percent) inquired about the probable cost of operation.

It can be noted that a large majority of the patients (80 percent reported that when they asked, the doctor provided the information about the cost involved. The percentage of patients having this viewpoint in government and private hospitals were 71.4 percent and 82.2 percent respectively.

Patients' Satisfaction about Care provided in Operation: Regarding the care provided during operation, a considerable majority of the patients (75 percent) reported satisfaction. But there was a significant difference in the satisfaction levels of patients of the government and private hospitals. Only a few patients (28.5 percent) of the government hospitals and a substantial majority of the patients (89 percent) of the private hospitals were satisfied with the care provided during the operation.

As regards, post-operative care, only 52.5 percent of patients were satisfied. Further, it can be observed that there is so much dissatisfaction in the patients of the government hospitals that an overwhelming majority of the patients (93 percent) expressed dissatisfaction with the post-operative care.

In the case of the private hospitals, a majority of the patients (67 percent) reported satisfaction with the post-operative care. Therefore, it seems that in this respect too the private hospitals are much better than the government hospitals.

4.3 Conclusion

The assessment of patients' perception of medical services has revealed dissatisfaction among the patients with the provision of medical services. Further, a significant difference has been found in the satisfaction level of male and female patients. Male patients were found to be more dissatisfied with quality of medical services in comparison to female patients.

The patients' satisfaction with the behaviour of the doctor and the hospital staff was also found to be significantly different among patients having different educational background. The graduate patients were found to be more dissatisfied in comparison to the patients having other qualifications.

It has also been found that the patients expressed dissatisfaction with the OPD services, stay in the hospital, care provided in the surgical operation and particularly, with the post-operative care. Further, the patients expressed dissatisfaction with the remedial measures adopted by hospitals in view of the complaints made by them.

Thus, the patients were found to be dissatisfied with the medical services. Although dissatisfied, not many patients expressed this openly as Indian patients hold doctors in high esteem.

The study has also revealed a wide communication gap between the doctor and the patients. Doctors were found to be lacking in providing information to the patients about the treatment given, options available, possible side-effects, risks involved, time required for recovery, causes of illness, future life style to be adopted and cost involved in the treatment. Further, the patients were found to be dissatisfied with the doctors' response towards their queries.

The improper behaviour of the doctor and the staff was found to be the major reason for the patients' dissatisfaction. However, it has been found that the patients go to a hospital which their doctor prescribes. The major reason for choosing a particular health institution was found to be the faith and popularity of the doctor. The major expectations of the patients from medical profession included immediate attention, proper diagnosis, sympathetic behaviour of doctor and reasonable charges.

Further, viewpoints of the majority of the patients reflect that some doctors are doing injustice to patients while performing their duties due to commercialisation of medical profession and doctors' not feeling the necessity of providing information about illness and treatment to the patients. However, the doctors in the government hospitals were also found to be overburdened with work and there were lack of proper facilities in those institutions.

The access of patients to redressal agencies under the CPA for redressal of their grievances against deficiency in medical services depends upon their awareness about the agencies under the CPA. The study has revealed that the level of patients' awareness about the Consumer Protection Act is not encouraging. Even some of the post-graduate and professionally qualified patients were found to be unaware of the CPA. Moreover, in a metropolitan city of Delhi where the accessibility to various mass media such as newspaper, television and radio is very high, it has been found that only a small number of patients (about 20 per cent) were aware about the Consumer Protection Act. There is a paramount need to increase the consumers' awareness about the various redressal agencies through the use of mass media.

Further, the study revealed that the dissatisfied patients wanted to take legal remedy under the CPA as they considered it to be speedier, cheaper and with minimum formalities in comparison to the Civil Courts. Thus, the patients have found the CPA to be beneficial to them in getting redressal of their grievances against deficiency in medical services.

Notes

1. "Law is Here to Serve the Public: An Interview with Justice V.B. Eradi", Health for the Millions (1992), December, Vol. 18, No. 6, p. 17.

Chapter 5

Grievance Redressal under Consumer Protection Act

This chapter is intended to examine the implications of application of the Consumer Protection Act (CPA) to medical services for the patient-doctor relationship. This is sought to be achieved by ascertaining the viewpoints of the doctors (from government and private health institutions and in private practice) and other knowledgeable persons under the 'expert' category which includes lawyers, judges, consumer activists from voluntary consumer organisations, journalists and professors of law.

It has been realised that there is a need for an independent and systematic study to ascertain the viewpoints of doctors and experts and also the difference in their opinion about the impact of the coverage of medical services under the CPA on the patient-doctor relationship and to determine whether the CPA would be beneficial to patients in getting redressal of their grievances against deficiency in medical services. Therefore, a survey of 60 doctors and 50 experts, including lawyers, judges, journalists, consumer activists and professors of law was conducted. The doctors were selected keeping in mind that they represent five major specialities, viz., medicine, surgery, obstetrics and gynaecology, paediatrics and orthopaedics. The survey was conducted through personal interview with the help of direct, structured and non-disguised questionnaires. The profile of such doctors and experts is presented below.

5.1 Profile of the Sample: Doctors

In order to ascertain the viewpoints of the doctors, it was decided to approach the doctors from all the major five specialities, viz., medicine, surgery, obstetrics and gynaecology, paediatrics, and orthopaedics. The doctors from both government and private health institutions were included. Twelve doctors from each speciality (8 from private and 4 from government hospitals) were approached, making the total number to 60. Due care was taken to include doctors having different demographic and behavioural characteristics. A profile of the sample of doctors on the basis of these characteristics is given in Table 5.1.

Age-wise distribution of the doctor respondents shows that a good number of doctors (45 percent) were in the category of 31 years to 50 years of age, while only 38.33 percent and 16.67 percent were in the category of more than 50 years and up to 30 years of age respectively.

Out of the total 60 doctors, 26 (43.33 percent) were males and 34 (56.67 percent) were females.

Education-wise, 25 (41.67 percent) doctors were M.B.B.S., while 35 (58.33 percent) doctors were post-graduate and above.

On the basis of occupation, 63.33 percent were reported to be in service, while 36.67 percent were in private practice.

As far as the area of specialisation is concerned, twelve doctors were approached from each major speciality in order to have representation of all the five major specialities, viz., medicine, surgery, obstetrics and gynaecology, paediatrics, and orthopaedics.

On the basis of professional experience, an equal number of doctors, 25 (41.67 percent), each had experience from 11 to 30 years and more than 30 years, while 10 doctors (16.67 percent) were in the category of up to 10 years of experience.

In order to have the viewpoints of doctors of both government and private health institutions, 20 doctors from government hospitals and 40 from private health institutions were approached. Since the CPA covers only the paid medical services, two-thirds of the doctors from private health institutions and one-third of doctors from government hospitals were included.

Table 5.1: Profile of Doctor-respondents

Demographic Characteristics	Doctor	
	Number	Percent
Distribution by Age:		
Upto 30 years	10	16.67
31 - 50 years	27	45.00
More than 50 years	23	38.33
Total	60	100.00
Distribution by sex:		
Male	26	43.33
Female	34	56.67
Total	60	100.00
Distribution by Education		
MBBS	25	41.57
Post-graduate & above	35	58.33
Total	60	100.00
Distribution by Occupation		
Service	38	63.33
Private Practice	22	36.67
Total	60	100.00
Distribution by Speciality		
Medicine	12	20.00
Surgery	12	20.00
Obstetrics & Gynaecology	12	20.00
Paediatrics	12	20.00
Orthopaedics	12	20.00
Total	60	100.00
Distribution by Professional Experience		
Upto 10 years	10	16.66
11 to 30 years	25	41.67
More than 30 years	25	41.67
Total	60	100.00
Distribution by Type of Health Institution		
Government Institutions	20	33.33
Private institutions	40	66.67
Total	60	100.00

5.2 Profile of the Sample: Experts

In order to ascertain the implications of application of the CPA to medical services for the patient-doctor relationship, experts' opinion was also sought. It was decided to approach the experts having varied areas of interest, including lawyers, judges, consumer activists from voluntary consumer organisations, journalists and professors of law having interest in the consumer protection laws. Care was also taken to include experts having different demographic and behavioural characteristics in order to have proper representation of each of these groups. A profile of the experts is presented in Table 5.2.

Table 5.2: Profile of Expert-respondents

Demographic Characteristics	Experts	
	Number	Percent
Distribution by Age:		
Upto 30 years	5	10
31 - 50 years	28	56
More than 50 years	17	34
Total	50	100
Distribution by sex:		
Male	35	70
Female	15	30
Total	50	100
Distribution by Education		
Graduate	15	30
Post-graduate & above	35	70
Total	50	100
Distribution by Occupation		
Service	31	62
Private Practice	19	38
Total	50	100
Distribution by Speciality		
Lawyer	15	30
Judges	3	6
Consumer activists	12	24
Journalists	15	30
Professor of Law	5	10
Total	50	100
Distribution by Professional Experience		
Upto 10 years	14	28
11 to 30 years	28	56
More than 30 years	8	16
Total	50	100

On the basis of age, 10 percent of the experts were up to 30 years of age, more than half of the experts (56 percent) were from 31 years to 50 years and the rest (34 percent) were more than 50 years of age.

Out of total 50 experts, 35 (70 percent) were male and 15 (30 percent) were female.

Education-wise, 30 percent were graduates, whereas a substantial majority of experts were post-graduates and above.

As regards the occupation, 62 percent of the expert-respondents were in service, while 38 percent were having their own practice.

In terms of the area of specialisation 30 percent were lawyers, 24 percent were consumer activists from voluntary consumer organisations, 30 percent were journalists, 6 percent were judges and 10 percent were professors of law.

Experience-wise, 28 percent of the experts were having professional experience up to 10 years, while more than half of the experts (56 percent) were having experience of 11 to 30 years and the rest (16 percent) were of more than 30 years of professional experience.

A look at the profile of both the doctors and the experts reveals that the sample is representative enough in the sense that respondents include representation of different age groups, education levels, occupations and areas of specialisation.

5.3 Viewpoints of the Doctors' and Experts About Medical Services

An analysis of the responses of the doctors and the experts is summarised in the following paragraphs.

5.3.1 Perceived Injustice to Patients by Doctors: A large majority of the doctors (63.3 percent) and an overwhelming majority of experts (90 percent) were of the view that some doctors were not doing justice to the patients while performing their duties (Table 5.3).

The major reasons advanced by the doctors for their not doing justice to the patients were: Lack of proper facilities (97.37 percent), overburdened with work (89.47 percent), doctors' not feeling the necessity to provide information to the patients (84.21 percent, and commercialisation (79.95 percent).

Table 5.3: Perceived Injustice to patients by Doctors

Particulars	No. of Respondents (per cent)			Experts
	Government	Private	Total	
	N=20	**N=40**	**N=60**	**N=50**
Some doctors are not doing justice towards their duties to patients	11 (55)	27 (67.5)	38 (63.3)	45 (90.0)
Possible causes of such injustice	**N=11**	**N=27**	**N=38**	**N=45**
Over burdened with work	11 (100)	23 (85.19)	34 (89.47)	14 (31.0)
Commercialisation	9 (81.81)	21 (77.78)	30 (78.95)	42 (93.3)
Resent being called at late hours	1 (9.09)	12 (44.44)	13 (34.21)	15 (33.3)
Lack of proper facilities	11 (100)	26 (96.30)	37 (97.37)	19 (42.2)
Doctors not feeling the necessity of providing information to patients	10 (90.90)	22 (81.48)	32 (84.21)	35 (77.7)

All the doctors (100 percent) of the government hospitals felt that the reasons for their not doing justice to the patients were two: they were overburdened with work and there were lack of proper facilities in the government hospitals.

As regards private hospitals, the reasons for not doing justice to the patients, besides the above mentioned two reasons were: commercialisation (77.78 percent) and the doctors' not feeling the necessity to provide information to the patients (81.48 percent).

Furthermore, the experts attributed commercialisation (93.3 percent) and doctors' not feeling necessity to provide information to the patients (77.7 percent) as the major reasons for doctors not doing justice to the patients. They suggested that doctor becoming a patients practice as followed in USA should also be implemented here. Wherein, doctors are admitted to hospital with a false name and a diagnosis and only the doctor admitting them really know who they really are to realise the difficulty and discomfort of hospitalised patients. This practice will give the doctor a better understanding of the state of mind of being a hospital patient and value of information provided to the patients.

5.3.2 Perception Regarding Doctors' Professional Accountability: A very large majority of doctors (76.6 percent) and an overwhelming majority of the experts (86 percent) were of the opinion that the doctors were accountable to some authority. Even those who opined that the doctors presently were not accountable, all (100 percent) felt that doctors should be accountable to some authority.

When asked to give their opinion about the authority to which doctors should be accountable, all the doctors (100 percent) opined in favour of the Medical Council of India and the Indian medical Association. While a whopping majority of the experts favoured the Consumer Court under the CPA (96 percent) and the Civil Court (94 percent).

5.3.3 Patients' Grievances against Doctors and Health Institutions: The major reasons advanced by the doctors and the experts for patients making complaint against doctors and health institutions are presented in Table 5.4.

The opinion of the doctors and experts did not differ much as far as the reasons for patients' dissatisfaction were concerned. The major reasons for patients' dissatisfaction advanced by the doctors and the experts were: Wrong diagnosis (63.3 percent and 74 percent respectively), unnecessary investigation (61.7 percent and 72 percent respectively) and negligence in informing patients about potentials risks and side-effects of prescribed drugs, procedure and tests (60 percent and 86 percent respectively).

Majority of the experts suggested that most of the problems arose out of a communication gap between the doctor and the patient. Therefore, the doctor should inform the patient about the provisional diagnosis, relevant investigations, necessary drugs prescribed, possible side-effects and the inherent risks in an operation, if recommended, and that too in a language understandable to the patient. Furthermore, they expressed that proper documentation and informed consent of the patients were necessary for a patient-doctor relationship. In addition, the experts considered lack of investigative facilities at the health institutions (52 percent) as the other major reason for patients' dissatisfaction.

Table 5.4: Patients Major Grievances against Doctors and Health Institutions

Major reasons for patients' dissatisfaction	No. of Respondents (percent)	
	Doctors N=60	Experts N=50
Non-availability of doctors when required	22 (36.7)	17 (34)
Non availability/inadequacy of other para medical service	27 (45.0)	20 (40)
Wrong diagnosis	38 (63.3)	37 (74)
Unnecessary Investigation	37 (61.7)	36 (72)
Over prescription	26 (43.3)	10 (20)
Lack of investigation facilities	21 (35.0)	26 (52)
Failure to advise hospitalisation when indicated by patient's condition	19 (31.7)	18 (36)
Negligence in informing patients of potential risks and side-effects of drugs and tests	36 (60.0)	43 (86)
Failure to obtain informed consent for procedures with inherent risks	13 (21.7)	9 (18)
Improper behaviour of the doctor	37 (61.7)	37 (74)
Improper behaviour of staff	28 (46.7)	34 (68)
Lack of general cleanliness in the premises	23 (38.3)	29 (58)
Overcharging	22 (36.7)	41 (82)
Patient instigated by other persons	30 (50.0)	9 (18)
For blackmailing	16 (26.7)	4 (8)
Patients' inability to judge doctor's expert opinion in terms of fees charged	46 (76.7)	21 (40)

Among the reasons for dissatisfaction of the patients, the doctors considered improper behaviour of the doctors (61.7 percent) and hospital staff (46.7 percent) as the main reasons, whereas, a vast majority of the experts (82 percent) opined that over-charging was the main cause for patients' dissatisfaction.

The other major reason responsible for dissatisfaction, in the opinion of both the doctors and the experts, was patient's inability to judge doctor's expert opinion in terms of fees charged.

5.3.4 Awareness about Avenues for Action against Deficiency in Medical Services: Awareness about various avenues available for action against deficiency in the medical services and also the avenue considered most appropriate by the doctors and the experts are shown in Table 5.5.

Table 5.5: Awareness about Avenues for Action against Deficiency in Medical Services

Avenues for action	No. of Respondents (Percent)			
	Awareness		Considered appropriate	
	Doctors N=60	Experts N=50	Doctors N=60	Experts N=50
Medical Council of India	54 (90.0)	50 (100)	34 (56.7)	8 (16.0)
State/Indian Medical Association	45 (75.0)	50 (100)	7 (11.7)	3 (6.0)
Civil Courts	58 (96.7)	50 (100)	9 (15.0)	4 (8.0)
CPA, 1986	51 (85.0)	50 (100)	10 (16.6)	35 (70.0)

It is clear from the Table 5.5 that a very large majority of doctors and all the experts were aware of various avenues, viz, the MCI, the IMA, the Civil Courts and the CPA, that are available for taking action against deficiency in medical services. More than half of the doctors (56.7 percent) and a few experts (16 percent) were in favour of the Medical Council of India. A substantial majority of experts (70 percent) considered the CPA as the most appropriate avenue for taking action. The doctors expressed that the medical technicalities of the case could be understood by medical experts, and that is why the MCI was considered as the most appropriate avenue. However, the experts felt that the CPA was a consumer welfare legislation and also comparatively more speedy, economical and with less formalities than the Civil Courts.

Further the experts expressed that since the Civil Courts were over-burdened with work and needed more procedural formalities, an ordinary patient could approach the CPA where it was easy to pursue the complaint. They also felt that people did not have much faith in the Medical Council of India and the State Medical Councils as these were mainly dominated by doctors. They were of the view that since the CPA kept the interest of both the doctors and the patients in mind and involved lesser number of technicalities, it was considered to be the most appropriate forum for the aggrieved patients. The doctors suggested that the Indian Medical Association should enlighten the consumer about the limitations of medical sciences and should take initiative to introduce medical audit system. The experts suggested that there was a need to educate about and make the general public aware of their rights as consumers and also about the avenues available for seeking redressal of their grievances.

5.3.5 Existing Legal Measures for Grievance Redressal: The opinion of the doctors and the experts about the existing legal measures available for redressal of patients' grievances which included the Law of Torts, the Indian Penal Code (IPC) and the Medical Council of India (MCI) is presented in Table 5.6.

Table 5.6: Existing Legal Measures for Redressal of Patients' Grievances

Particulars	No. of Respondents (Percent)	
	Doctors	Experts
Existing legal measures considered sufficient to provide redressal against deficiency in medical services	15 (25)	4 (8)
Existing legal measures considered not sufficient to provide redressal against deficiency in medical services	45 (75)	46 (92)
Total	60 (100)	50 (100)

A considerable majority of doctors (75 percent) and a whopping majority of experts (92 percent) were of the opinion that the existing legal measures including the Law of Torts, the Indian Penal Code and the Indian Medical Council Act were not sufficient to provide redressal to the patients against deficiency in medical services. Their opinion regarding the most appropriate step to be taken is shown in Table 5.7.

Table 5.7: Most Appropriate Step to Get Redressal of Patients' Grievances

Step to be taken	No. of Respondents (percent)	
	Doctors N=45	Experts N = 46
The MCI should be made more powerful so as to provide compensation to aggrieved patients	20 (44.4)	10 (20.0)
Redressal should be sought under the CPA in its present form	2 (4.4)	21 (42.0)
Amendments in the CPA should be made to include expert from medical field	20 (44.4)	12 (24.0)
Civil laws be made more speedier and cheaper	6 (13.3)	4 (8.0)

Regarding the most appropriate step to be taken, a good number of doctors (44.4 percent) opined for the IMC Act to be made more powerful to provide compensation and some amendment in the CPA to be made to include medical expert. The doctors suggested that the MCI should take stern action against the doctors who were not performing their duties up to a reasonable level of quality so that the patients feel attracted to the MCI for their grievance redressal. Further, they suggested that evaluation of performance of a medical practitioner should be done by the MCI, every five years and the licence be renewed only after its satisfaction. However, a good number of experts (42 percent) were of the view that redressal should be sought under the CPA in its present form. Thus, the opinion of the doctors and the experts are quite different on this aspect. The experts suggested that the CPA would be beneficial to patients, if implemented properly with good infrastructure, therefore, steps should be taken by the government to improve implementation of the CPA otherwise like the Civil Courts, the Consumer Courts would also be overburdened with work and the faith in the Consumer Courts would also get eroded. Further, they suggested that voluntary consumer organisations should take up the task of informal reconciliation, whereby, litigation would be minimised.

5.3.6 Perception Regarding Inclusion of Free Medical Services under CPA: Perception of the doctors and the experts regarding the inclusion of free medical services under the Consumer Protection Act 1986, is shown in Table 5.8. As shown in the Table, some doctors (25 percent) and an overwhelming majority of experts (90 percent) were of the view that the free medical services provided by the government hospitals and other health institutions should also be covered under the CPA. The doctors expressed that negligence has to be taken care of, whether paid or not; the poor patients should get proper justice and compensation for the loss. Further, services should be treated at par and there should not be any disparity between free medical service and paid medical service. Furthermore, both the doctors and the experts felt that with inclusion of free service, doctors in the government hospitals would become more vigilant and would impart medical information to the patients in a more responsible and sincere manner.

Table 5.8: Perception regarding Inclusion of Free Medical Services under the CPA

Particulars	No. of Respondents (percent)	
	Doctors	Experts
Should free service provided by government hospitals and other health institutions be covered under the CPA?		
Yes	15 (25)	45 (90)
No	45 (75)	5 (10)
Total	60 (100)	50 (100)

The experts gave the viewpoint that if there was negligence or deficiency in rendering medical service to patients which resulted in loss, then irrespective of charges, patients must be compensated and for this the Act needed to be amended to include free service. Furthermore, they expressed that negligence should be treated and compensated at par whether paid or not and patients should get proper justice without any disparity. They felt that what decided the patient-doctor relationship was not the money that the patients spent but it was the treatment they got from the doctors. They expressed that accountability had to be there and payment of fees should be no consideration for compensating aggrieved patients.

Some experts opined that if free services provided by government hospitals were included, then doctors would become more vigilant, careful and responsible and would be more diligent and sincere in attending patients.

Further, some of the experts felt that as people were paying taxes which was the indirect payment for free services, and otherwise also, poor patients should not suffer and should be allowed to get compensation for deficiency in medical services. They expressed that most of the complaints of negligence were reported from the government hospitals, therefore, the government hospitals and doctors providing free services should not be spared for negligence and they should be held accountable for their acts of misconduct and negligence. Some of the experts felt that as the doctors were dealing with life, which was the most precious thing, the need for ensuring reasonable standard of patient-care was equally necessary in the government hospitals providing free medical services. Further, they felt that the charges for the service was a separate and secondary issue which could not be the absolute basis for judging the quality of patient-care and moreover, proven negligence of the doctors should be penalised and aggrieved patients should get compensation. According to Mr. H. D. Shourie, Convenor, Common Cause, the segregation done by the Supreme Court by not covering free government health institutions and charitable institutions was wrong. He further opined that in near future consumer activists should move to the Court to demand that all doctors be brought under the purview of the CPA [1].

The Voluntary Health Association of India (VHAI) also expressed deep concern over non-inclusion of free government health institutions under the purview of the CPA. The VHAI felt that majority of the poor patients would not be able to avail themselves of benefits of the CPA [2].

5.3.7 Perception Regarding Redressal Mechanism under the CPA: The opinion of the doctors and the experts regarding the redressal mechanism under the CPA is presented in Table 5.9. As shown in Table, a large majority of doctors (63.88 percent) and an overwhelming majority of experts (80.66 percent) were of the opinion that in comparison to the Civil Courts, the redressal under the CPA was speedy, inexpensive and involved minimum formalities. Thus, both the doctors and the experts expressed the same opinion on this aspect.

Table 5.9: Perception Regarding Redressal Mechanism under the CPA

Particulars	No. of Respondents (percent)	
	Doctors N = 60	Experts N = 50
In comparison to the Civil Courts, the redressal under the CPA is :		
Speedy	37.00 (61.67)	40.00 (80.00)
Inexpensive	39.00 (65.00)	42.00 (84.00)
With minimum formalities	39.00 (65.00)	39.00 (78.00)
Mean (X)	38.33 (63.88)	40.33 (80.66)

5.3.8 Perception regarding Basis of Patient-Doctor Relationship: A summary of the views of the doctors and the experts regarding the patient-doctor relationship is presented in Table 5.10. It can be observed from the Table that an overwhelming majority of the doctors (91.67 percent) and a good majority of experts (60 percent) believed that the relationship between patient and doctor was that of mutual trust and faith. They observed that for this the patients should be told frankly about the possibilities of the treatment and the doctors should encourage proper communication with the patients. however, a good number of experts (40 percent) felt that the relationship was a mere contract where the patient is a weaker party. None of the doctors expressed this viewpoint.

Table 5.10: Perception Regarding Basis of Patient-Doctor Relationship

Particulars	Respondents			
	Doctors		Experts	
	Number	Percent	Number	Percent
Patient-doctor relationship is based on:				
Trader and Buyer	5	8.33		
Mutual trust and faith	55	91.67	30	60
Master and servant	--	--	--	--
Contract where both the patients can decide freely	--	--	--	--
Contract where the patient is a weaker party	--	--	20	40
Total	60	100	50	100

5.3.9 Effect of CPA on Patient-Doctor Relationship: As shown in Table 5.11, a large majority of doctors (68.33 percent) opined that the patient-doctor relationship would deteriorate with the coverage of medical services under the CPA. The reason given by doctors was that the treatment would become much more expensive as doctors would resort to defensive medical practices, including ordering of more investigations in order to play safe. Further, they expressed that faith would be lost in the relationship and the doctors would start suspecting patients as potential litigants. however, a few doctors (13.33 percent) opined that the relationship would improve as doctors would become more careful towards their duties.

It can be observed from Table 5.11 that the experts were divided on this issue. 34 percent of the experts were of the opinion that the relationship would deteriorate whereas 36 percent believed that it would improve. The experts who were of the view that the relationship would deteriorate felt that as the CPA was implemented on the patient-doctor relationship, initially, for some period, the mutual faith and trust would be lost, the gap between the patient and the doctor would increase and doctors would resort to defensive medical practices. The experts who advocated that the relationship would improve gave the viewpoint that doctors would become more careful towards their duties for fear of being sued, if found negligent. Further, they felt that doctors would become more conscious of their responsibilities towards patients and patients awareness towards their rights would increase.

Table 5.11: Effect of CPA on Patient-doctor Relationship

Particulars	Respondents			
	Doctors		Experts	
	Number	Percent	Number	Percent
As the CPA is implemented on medical services, the patient-doctor relationship would:				
Deteriorate	41	68.34	17	34
Not affected	11	18.33	13	26
Improve	8	13.33	18	36
Total	60	100.00	50	100

Another 26 percent of the experts felt that the patient-doctor relationship would not be affected in the long-run. They opined that it was only in the short-run that the doctors would be getting furious. Moreover, they felt that Indian patients would not unnecessarily harm the doctors. Further, they expressed that with the passage of time, there would not be any fear among doctors and doctors would treat patients in the best possible manner. Thus, in the long run, relationship would not be affected as the short-run effects would get neutralised.

5.3.10 Effect of CPA on Quality of Medical Services: The opinion of the doctors and the experts regarding the effect of the

CPA on the quality of medical services provided to patients is shown in Table 5.12.

A large majority of doctors (70 percent) and a very large majority of the experts (86 percent) were of the opinion that the quality of medical services would improve with the coverage of medical services under the CPA. Thus, both the doctors and the experts held the same view on this aspect. Only a few doctors (16.7 percent) and a negligible number of experts (4 percent) opined that the quality of medical service would deteriorate to some extent, while none of the doctors and experts felt that it would deteriorate drastically. Therefore, coverage of the medical services under CPA would result in improvement in the quality of services provided to the patients by the doctors and health institutions.

Table 5.12: Effect of CPA on Quality of Medical Services

Particulars	Respondents			
	Doctors		Experts	
	Number	Percent	Number	Percent
As the CPA is implemented to medical services, the quality of service provided by doctor and health institution would:				
Improve tremendously	5	8.3	7	14
Improve to some extent	37	61.7	36	72
Not affected	8	13.3	4	8
Deteriorate to some extent	10	16.7	2	4
Deteriorate drastically	--	--	--	--
Total	60	100.0	50	100.0

5.3.11 Implications of Application of CPA to Medical Services for Patient-doctor Relationship: In order to examine the implications of application of the CPA to medical services for the patient-doctor relationship, opinion of the doctors and the experts was sought on various aspects including social, ethical, economic, and related to medical education and profession, that would likely to affect provision of medical services to patients and the patient-doctor relationship. The major findings of their responses are presented here.

As the patients' awareness towards their right to quality medical care is concerned, a substantially large majority of doctors (85 percent) and an overwhelming large majority of experts (92 percent) opined that it would increase.

More than half of the doctors (58.3 percent) and a very large number of the experts (70 percent) were of the opinion that the patients would be in a better position to bargain for better medical care. Furthermore, both the doctors (95 percent) and the experts (90 percent) in a whopping majority expressed that the doctor would become more careful in performance of his duties towards the patient.

Majority of the doctors (60 percent) responded that with the coverage of the medical services under the CPA, doctors would start seeing every patient as a potential litigant. however, majority of the experts (62 percent) did not confirm this view. It implies that the opinion of the doctors and the experts differs on this aspect.

Again, the opinion of the doctors and the experts differs regarding the patients becoming litigation-minded after the implementation of the CPA on medical services. Majority of the doctors (65 percent) confirmed this view, while substantial majority of the experts (72 percent) did not express this viewpoint.

Regarding the patients and their relatives accusing doctors for every adverse outcome, while a majority of the doctors (65 percent) opined this viewpoint, majority of the experts (60 percent) did not respond to this. Thus, again their viewpoints differ on this aspect.

A large majority of doctors (81.7 percent) and a good majority of experts (66 percent) were of the view that in the absence of screening of complaints before initiating proceedings, there was more likelihood of vexatious complaints. Thus, both the doctors and the experts hold the same viewpoint on this aspect.

More than half of the doctors (58.3 percent) felt that doctors would become an easy subject of blackmailing, while a substantial majority of the experts (70 percent) did not hold this view. Thus, the opinion of the doctors and the experts differs on this aspect too.

Regarding the possibility of lawyers and patients conniving together to blackmail doctors, a good majority of the doctors (76.7 percent) confirmed this view, whereas there were only a few experts (38 percent) who held this view.

Both the doctors (91.7 percent) and the experts (74 percent) in large majority felt that litigation against doctors would adversely affect their reputation irrespective of the result of litigation. They further opined that the cases against doctors should not be published unless negligence was proved.

A large majority of the doctors (78.3 percent) and the experts (70 percent) felt that doctors would hesitate in attending to emergency cases. Similarly, a majority of doctors (60 percent) and experts (60 percent) held the opinion that doctors would become hesitant in attending to serious patients. Thus, both the doctors and experts had shown agreement on these aspects.

A large majority of the doctors (76 percent) responded that the doctors would hesitate in using risky procedures and drugs even in emergencies, while only a few experts (44 percent) held this viewpoint.

Less than half of the doctors (45 percent) and very few experts (14 percent) opined that in future doctors might not like to work in 'high risk' areas such as obstetrics and neuro-surgery.

As far as practice of defensive medicine was concerned, both the doctors (85 percent) and the experts (74 percent) in large majority felt that doctors would start practising defensive medicine such as ordering more investigations just to play safe.

Both doctors (69.7 percent) and the experts (66.8 percent) in a large majority were of the view that the doctor would suffer monetary loss because of adverse effect on reputation in the form of reduced number of patients, money spent in defending cases, money lost due to not seeing patients as most of the time would be spent in defending cases, money paid as compensation and as insurance premium.

An overwhelming majority of the doctors (95 percent) and the experts (96 percent) opined that doctors would take insurance policies. Some of the doctors declared that they had already taken them. Again, a substantial majority of the doctors (91.7 percent) and the experts (88 percent) responded that the doctor would start ordering more investigations just to play safe. It implies that patients will have to pay more for medical treatment.

In response to the query about the effect of coverage of medical services under the CPA on the cost of health care, a whopping majority of respondents in both the categories: doctors (96.6 percent) and experts (94 percent) opined that the cost of medical treatment would increase. Further they opined that it might become unaffordable to the people belonging to lower middle class.

Thus, both the doctors and the experts felt that the coverage of medical services under the CPA would lead to the increase in the cost of health care.

A substantial majority of the doctors (73.3 percent) and a good majority of experts (60 percent) felt that the doctors would start taking their training and education more seriously.

A very large majority of both the doctors (86.7 percent) and the experts (74 percent) expressed that with the coverage of medical services under the CPA doctors would try to update their knowledge and become more careful. Again, an overwhelming majority of the doctors (91.7 percent) and a very large majority of the experts (86 percent) confirmed the view that doctors would start maintaining adequate records of their patients.

From the above analysis of the responses, it appears that the coverage of medical services under the CPA would lead to improvement in the quality of treatment provided by doctors and health institutions.

In order to ascertain whether there is a significant difference in the opinion of the doctors and the experts regarding the implications of the CPA for the patient-doctor relationship, t-test for all the implications was calculated.

There appears to be a highly significant difference in the opinion of the doctors and the experts regarding the implications of the CPA for the patient-doctor relationship. The doctors seemed to view that with the coverage of medical services under the CPA, the cost of treatment would increase, doctors would start practising defensive medicine which included ordering every possible investigations to confirm the diagnosis and doctors would start seeing patients as potential litigants and consequently would hesitate in seeing serious patients. However, the experts did not view these as the possible implications. They expressed that these were only short-run apprehensions of the doctors which would not affect patient-doctors relationship in the long run. In their opinion, the patient-doctor relationship in the long run would remain on the basis of mutual faith and trust.

5.3.12 Perception Regarding CPA's Role in Grievance Redressal of Patients: The opinion of the doctors and the experts was sought on whether the applicability of the CPA to the medical services would be helpful to patients in getting their grievances redress. Their responses are shown in Table 5.13.

Table 5.13: Perception Regarding CPA's Role in Grievance Redressal of Patients

Particulars	Respondents			
	Doctors		Experts	
	Number	Percent	Number	Percent
The CPA would be helpful to patients in getting redressal of their grievances:				
Yes	25	42	42	94
No	35	58	8	16
Total	60	100	50	100

A good number of the doctors (42 percent) and an

overwhelming majority of the experts (94 percent) were of the opinion that the Consumer Protection Act, 1986 would be beneficial to patients in getting the redressal of their grievances against deficiency in medical services. however, more than half of the doctors (58 percent) held a contrary view on this aspect.

5.3.13 Doctors' Views on Additional Aspects: The opinion of the doctors about the patients' expectations from the medical profession, necessity of continuing medical education and maintenance of patients' records was sought. The summary of the findings is presented below.

Patients' Expectations from Medical Profession: 'Immediate attention' was ranked first which implies that in the doctors' opinion, the patients expect immediate attention from the doctors. In addition to immediate attention, other major expectations of the patients according to doctors include: proper diagnosis, thorough examination, quick relief and doctors' sympathetic behaviour.

More than half of the doctors (56.67 percent) did not view more information about illness to patients' as the main expectation as they have ranked it the last.

Necessity of Continuing Medical Education: Doctors' opinion about the necessity of continuing medical education and the actions taken by the doctors to update their knowledge is presented in Table 5.14.

All the doctors expressed that continuing medical education was necessary for the practising doctors. An overwhelming majority of the doctors (85 percent) opined that doctors should subscribe to medical journals for updating their knowledge. A substantial majority of the doctors also expressed that doctors should attend professional seminars and conferences (70 percent) and participate in training programmes (75 percent) in order to update their knowledge. They suggested that continuous education and development be provided including a refresher course through the powerful medium like Television.

Table 5.14: Necessity of Continuing Medical Education

Statements	Doctors (N = 60)	
	Number	Percent
Continuing medical education is necessary for practising doctors	60	100
Continuing medical education is not necessary for practising doctors	Nil	Nil
For updating knowledge doctors should:		
Subscribe to medical journals	51	85
Attend professional conferences and seminars	42	70
Participate in training programmes	45	75
Watch pertinent video films	10	17

Maintenance of Patients' Records: As shown in Table 5.15, more than half the number of doctors (51.6 percent) reported that they maintained adequate patients' record. However, quite a large number (48.4 percent) also expressed that they did not maintain elaborate patients' records. When asked, whether they had started maintaining elaborate records after the implementation of the CPA, a substantially large majority of the doctors (80 percent) opined in favour of the question. Thus, with the implementation of the CPA, doctors have become more careful and have started maintaining adequate patients' records.

Table 5.15: Maintenance of Patients' Records

Particulars	Doctors (N = 60)	
	Number	Percent
Do doctors maintain adequate patients' record?		
Yes	31	51.6
No	29	48.4
After the coverage of medical services under the CPA, have the doctors started maintaining elaborate records?		
Yes	48	80.0
No	12	20.0

5.4 Conclusion

The analysis of the viewpoints of the doctors and experts has revealed that some doctors are not doing justice to the patients while performing their duties. The major reasons, were found to be commercialisation and doctors' not feeling the necessity to provide information about illness and treatment to the patients. Further, the doctors in the government hospitals were found to be overburdened with work and there were lack of proper facilities in the health institutions.

Improper behaviour of the doctor and the staff and lack of communication on the part of the doctors about the treatment, possible side-effects and risks were found to be the major reasons for patients' dissatisfaction in the opinion of the doctors and the experts.

The awareness of the doctors and the experts about the avenues available for redressal of grievances against deficiency in medical services were found to be high. The Medical Council of India was considered to be the best avenue by the doctors, while, the Consumer Protection Act was favoured by the experts.

Further, both the doctors and the experts found legal measures including the law of Torts, the Indian Penal Code and the Indian Medical Council (IMC) Act, not sufficient to provide speedy redressal to patients. The most appropriate step in the doctors' opinion was to amend the IMC Act to provide compensation or to amend the CPA to include medical expert. However, the experts favoured the Consumer protection Act, 1986, in its present form as a means of redressal for patients as they considered it to be speedier, economical and with minimum formalities in comparison to the Civil Courts. Further, the study has revealed that the free medical services should also be included under the CPA.

The study has shown that the patient-doctor relationship is based on mutual trust and faith. However, some experts also considered it to be a relationship where patients was a weaker party. Further, majority of the doctors opined that with the coverage of medical services under the CPA, the patient-doctor relationship might get adversely affected as doctors had started practising defensive medicine which included ordering unnecessary investigations just to play safe and started buying insurance policies whereby making the treatment costly for patients. however, experts opined that patient-doctor relationship though might get adversely affected in the short-run because of above mentioned reasons, would not be affected in the long-run. They expressed that the short-run effects would get neutralised in the long-run. Further, they opined that with the coverage of medical services under the CPA, the doctors would become more careful towards their duties, thereby improving their relationship with the patients.

It has also been found that all the doctors were feeling the necessity of continuing medical education to update their knowledge. It has been found that doctors understands patients' expectations which included immediate attention, proper diagnosis and sympathetic behaviour of the doctor.

The study has also shown that the doctors were not maintaining adequate patients' records but the enforcement of the regulatory measures under the CPA in relation to medical services would prompt them to maintain proper patients' records.

The study has revealed a significant difference in the opinion of the doctors and the experts regarding the implications of the CPA for the patient-doctor relationship. While the doctors felt that both doctors and patients would start suspecting each other and because of practice of defensive medicine which included ordering every possible investigation and insurance policies taken up by the doctors, the cost of treatment would increase. It has also been found that there would be hesitation on the part of the doctors in attending to serious and emergency patients. However, experts did not show agreement in these regards.

Further, the study has indicated that patients' awareness about their rights to quality medical care would increase, thus making doctors more careful in performing their duties. Further, the application of the CPA would make doctors more careful towards their training and education, in up-dating their knowledge and in maintaining patients' records.

It can be concluded that a large majority of experts and a good number of doctors found the CPA to be beneficial to patients in getting their grievances redressed. However, doctors also felt that application of CPA would lead to substantial increase in the cost of treatment.

Notes

1. As quoted in Sharma, Anju (1995), "Divergent Views on Verdict on Doctors", The Hindustan Times, November 16.

2. The Hindustan Times (1995), "S.C. Verdict is Incomplete", November 16.

Chapter 6

Conclusions

This chapter consolidates the major conclusions of the study.

6.1 Approach of Consumer Courts under CPA

The study has shown that there is substantial increase in the number of complaints received and appeals filed relating to deficiency in medical services after the landmark judgement of the Supreme Court in the case of *Indian Medical Association vs. V.P. Shantha*, delivered in 1995. Further, the disposal rate of complaints by the National Consumer Disputes Redressal Commission and the Delhi State Consumer Disputes Redressal Commission was found to be 56.83 percent and 63.83 per cent respectively, upto March 31, 2001, which implies that 43.17 percent and 36.17 percent complaints respectively, are still pending before these Courts.

From the review of the cases decided by the National Commission and various state commissions set up under the Consumer Protection Act, 1986, it can be concluded that the Consumer Courts have conducted themselves judiciously and that they have taken both letter and spirit of the law into account. The study has shown that with the landmark judgement of the Supreme Court in the case of *Indian Medical Association v. V.P. Shantha*, delivered in 1995, the awareness and confidence of the patients in the grievances redressal system under the Consumer Protection Act, 1986 has considerably increased. There has been a substantial increase in the number of complaints received and appeals field in the cases relating to deficiency in medical services after the judgement of the apex Court.

The attitude of the Consumer Courts towards aggrieved patients has been favourable. However, it is not always that the verdict of the Consumer Courts have gone in favour of the patient, they have also dismissed a number of complaints where the complainant failed to prove negligence on the part of doctor or health institution. The Consumer Courts have also taken strict actions against those patients who had filed frivolous or vexatious complaints just to humiliate the doctors. Thus, the redressal machinery under the Consumer Protection Act, 1986 has provided justice to both the patients and the doctors. Further, the adjudicating agencies under the CPA offer sufficient guarantee of justice to both patients and doctors as the provision of appeals and revisions are also provided under the Consumer Protection Act, 1986.

Thus, Consumer Courts have shown that the law is not against the honest and well-meaning doctors. In the cases, where the complainant tried to blackmail or humiliate the doctor by filing a frivolous or vexatious complaint, the Consumer Courts have taken a serious view and penalised the complainant by imposing maximum possible penalty prescribed under the Act. Thus, the redressal machinery under the Consumer Protection Act has proved to be a protector for those patients who pay for their services and also provide necessary protection to the doctors and health institutions against malafide litigations.

Out of the 53 cases reviewed in the present study which were decided by the National Commission upto January 31, 2001, 24.53 percent were decided in favour of patients. In 60.38 percent of the cases the National Commission did not find any deficiency on the part of the doctor or the health institution in providing the medical services. The National Commission also remanded back to the State Commissions, six cases for giving opportunities to both parties to produce more evidences.

In the cases of frivolous or vexatious complaints, the National Commission also provided costs to complainants. Even the maximum amount of Rs. 10,000 (under Section 26 of the CPA) was considered by the National Commission to be on the lower side to compensate the doctor who had faced so much humiliation.

From the review of 225 cases decided by various State Commissions till January 31, 2001, it was observed that 24 percent cases were decided in favour of the patients. However, in 64.89 percent cases, negligence on the part of the doctor or the health institution was not proved.

Further, death was not found to be the cause for filing complaints against doctors and health institutions (in 60.38 percent of the cases decided by the National Commission and in 72 percent of the cases decided by various state Commissions). However, complaints were largely related to deficiency in surgical treatment as against non-surgical treatment (in 62.26 percent of the cases decided by the National Commission and in 53.78 percent of the cases decided by various State Commissions).

Regarding fees charged by the doctors, it was upheld by the Haryana State Commission that a doctor can fix his fees since there is no yard stick to fix up any uniform scale of fees so that it is found to differ from one doctor to another. Further, the Tamil Nadu State Commission has made it clear that the health institution cannot be made vicariously liable for the negligent act of the doctor when the doctor is paying rent to the hospital for using the space.

The time taken by the Consumer Courts in deciding the complaints and appeals was found to be quite long. In certain cases, the National Commission took as long as four years in deciding a case. In the initial years of functioning, there was no case left pending for disposal with the National Commission and various State Commissions. However, from the year 1992, the number of cases pending for disposal have increased at a very fast rate so much so that more than 40 percent cases were pending till March 31, 2001, in the National Commission and in various State Commissions. The position of the Delhi State Commission is virtually the same, where 36.17 percent cases were pending for disposal for the same period.

This undue delay tends to defeat the purpose of providing

speedy remedy to aggrieved consumers. The study found that the delay is mainly due to lack of personnel and other resources with the Consumer Courts. With the increase in their work-load, their financial and other resources have also to be augmented. The grievance redressal system under the Consumer Protection Act would be beneficial to the patients, if the Act is implemented properly with good infrastructure. For this, it is imperative that necessary institutional infrastructure must be provided as envisaged under the Act.

Therefore, steps should be taken by the government to improve implementation of redressal mechanism under the CPA, otherwise, like the Civil Courts, the Consumer Courts would also be overburdened and faith in the Consumer Courts would get eroded.

Furthermore, as felt by the National Commission also, the amount of Rs. 10,000 as cost against the person making a frivolous or vexatious complaint is inadequate. It is suggested that the provision in Section 26 of the Consumer Protection Act, 1986, be amended so as to provide deterrent punishment against misuse of the statutory measures of consumer protection by unscrupulous people. In a case where it is established that the complaint is not only false and vexatious but also that it has been filed with the intention of blackmailing the doctor, the Forums should be empowered to award substantive sentence of imprisonment to the complainant so that the consumer is discouraged from resorting to frivolous proceedings.

It is also suggested that before the final decision of the case, no publicity relating to it be allowed. The reputation of the doctors in their profession matters a lot to them which can be adversely affected by these false, baseless or vexatious complaints. The mere filing of complaint can cause irreparable damage to the fair name and respect of the doctor, though, ultimately nothing may come out of it. The damage (the maximum being Rs.10,000 as contemplated under Section 26 of the CPA, 1986) which is awarded to the doctor, is no substitute of the harassment and ignominy of trials under the CPA that he has gone through, especially where the motive is to blackmail or to coerce the doctor to pay something.

6.2 Patients' Perception of Medical Services and Grievance Redressal under CPA

6.2.1 Patients' Satisfaction with Medical Services: The study has revealed that patients were not much satisfied with medical services provided to them by doctors and health institutions. Regarding the patients' satisfaction about the quality of services provided by health institutions at various levels including reception, administration, cleanliness, nursing staff, doctors, investigations, supply of written records and medical store, the study revealed a significant difference in the opinion of the male and female patients. Female patients were found to be more satisfied in comparison to male. The study also showed that the satisfaction level of the patients of government and private health institutions differ significantly. Patients of the private health institutions were found to be more satisfied in comparison to the patients of the government hospitals. However, patients' satisfaction does not differ significantly among patients having different educational background and patients having different age groups.

Patients' Satisfaction with Behaviour of Doctor and Hospital Staff: Regarding the behaviour of doctors, nurses, and other para-medical staff, the patients' satisfaction was found to be significantly different among patients having different educational background. While illiterate patients were found to be satisfied, the graduate patients tended to be dissatisfied.

The study also found highly significant difference in patients' satisfaction of government and private health institutions as far as the behaviour of doctors and other hospital staff was concerned. The patients of private health institutions were found to be much more satisfied in comparison to the patients of government hospitals.

Patients' Satisfaction with OPD Services: The study has revealed that the patients of government hospitals have to wait much longer for the doctor than the patients of private hospitals. While the average waiting time for the doctor in government hospitals was found to be more than one hour, it was upto half an hour in private hospitals.

As regards the performance of staff at the registration counter, the study has shown that majority of patients found the staff of government hospitals inefficient and unconcerned. However, the staff of private hospitals were found to be efficient and helpful.

Regarding the time spent by the doctor in examining the patients, the patients have stated that the doctors do not generally spend enough time (only up to 5 minutes) to examine a patient.

However, the necessary facilities including X-ray, CT-scan and ECG were found to be displayed at the counter in both government and private hospitals.

Patients' Satisfaction during their Stay in the Health Institution: On the aspects relating to admission and stay in the health institutions, the study has shown that the patients were not much satisfied. While the average waiting time for admission was found to be unduly long in the government hospitals, it was reasonable in the private hospitals.

As regards the display of rates of charges for medical services, the study has shown that majority of the patients found these to be displayed at the appropriate places.

Further, the study has shown that the patients of the government hospitals were attended, on arrival in the ward by a nurse after at least half an hour and by a junior and a senior doctor after one hour. However, the majority of the patients of private hospitals have stated that a nurse arrived within 10 minutes and a junior and a senior doctor within half an hour.

Thus, the private health institutions were found to be somewhat more efficient than the government health institutions.

Patients' Satisfaction with Care Provided in Surgical Operation: The opinion of the patients who had undergone surgery has reflected that the doctors do not generally provide the adequate information about the operation to be undergone. Majority of the patients of both government and private health institutions, who had undergone some surgical operation expressed that the doctor only told them that the operation would be done but did not explain them about the line of treatment, risks involved, and the future life style to be adopted before taking their consent.

The study has further shown that the information about the cost involved in the operation was provided only when the patients asked for it.

As regards the patients' satisfaction with the care provided during and after the operation, the study has shown a contrast in the opinion of the patients of government and private health institutions. Majority of the patients of the government hospitals expressed dissatisfaction with the care provided during an operation and especially with the post-operative care. The patients of the private hospitals, however, expressed satisfaction with the care. Furthermore, the number of patients dissatisfied with post-operative care were more than the number of patients dissatisfied with care provided during operation in the case of both government and private health institutions. Thus, the health institutions are lacking in providing post-operative care to the patients.

The study has shown that the patients felt dissatisfied with the services provided at the out-patient department (OPD), stay in the hospitals, care provided during surgical operation and particularly with the post-operative care. Furthermore, the patients expressed dissatisfaction with the remedial measures adopted by the health institutions in response to their complaints.

Although the patients were found to be dissatisfied with the medical services provided, not many expressed this openly when asked about the extent of their overall satisfaction or otherwise, regarding the provision of medical services. This is because, the Indian patients, generally do not like to speak against the medical profession which enjoys high esteem in the minds of the general public.

6.2.2 Reasons for Patients' Dissatisfaction: The improper behaviour of the doctor and the hospital staff was found to be the main reason for patients' dissatisfaction. The opinion of the patients, doctors and experts clearly reflects that the doctors are not doing justice to their patients while performing their duties. The major reasons included : commercialisation of medical profession and the doctors not feeling the necessity to provide information to the patients about their illness and the line of treatment. However, the doctors in government hospitals were found to be overburdened with work and these hospitals were found to be lacking in proper facilities.

Thus, it appears that doctors are becoming more and more commercialised and the ethical norms as encoded in the 'Code of Medical Ethics' by the Medical Council of India are rarely adhered to. It is, therefore, suggested that a paper on 'medical ethics and liability and accountability for medical negligence' should be taught at the undergraduate level to medical students, so that they enhance their knowledge on such a relevant subject. Moreover, the Medical Council of India should take strong steps to effectively implement the code so that it is taken seriously by both the doctors and the patients.

As improper behaviour of the doctors and hospital staff was found to be the main irritant for the patients and the study has revealed that doctors were not doing justice to patients, it has become necessary that 'medical audit system' should be adopted by the hospitals in both the private and the public sectors for facilitating self-assessment and comparing with set standards of medical care, based on patients' expectations, so that the deficiency in services can be detected and corrected and thereby an improvement in patient care is brought about.

Since the patients felt dissatisfied with remedial measures adopted by the hospital authorities in relation to their complaints, the concept of 'quality control circle' can be adopted by the health institutions as has been successfully adopted by the State Bank of India to involve employees at each level to solve consumer problems, or 'ombudsman' can be created in health institutions as has been successfully functioning in the leading newspaper, The Times of India, to provide speedy and effective redressal of patients' complaints. The health care institutions separately or collectively or the Indian Medical Association on their behalf can set up ombudsman to redress patients' grievances. The service of the ombudsman can be useful to those consumers who are reluctant to take legal remedy. By this system, the burden on the legal system can be reduced.

Further, the 'patients' charter', prepared by the Ministry of Civil Supplies, Consumer Affairs and Public Distribution, which sets out basic standards for health facilities and rights and duties of doctors and patients should be implemented properly. The charter is only a tool to increase awareness about the need to protect some basic principles. It is not an end in itself, but merely another step in the strategy to put into practice the principles it contains. Therefore, it is suggested that proper steps should be taken by the Ministry to effectively implement the 'patients' charter' for health services.

6.2.3 Communication of Information about Line of Treatment: The study has indicated wide communication gap between the doctor and the patients. The study has shown that the doctor do not spend enough time but only up to 5 minutes in examining the patients and do not explain them about the treatment, options available, possible side-effects and complications, unforeseen consequences and risks involved, time required for recovery, future life style to be adopted and the cost involved in the treatment and the operation.

The study has also shown that majority of the patients felt that they ought to be told about the line of treatment, and therefore they should insist on the doctors' informing them of this. Further, the study has revealed that as the education level becomes higher, the percentage of patients actually asking the doctor about the line of treatment increases. The study has also shown that all the post-graduate and professionally qualified patients actually asked the doctor about their line of treatment. However, out of such patients majority of them were found to be dissatisfied with doctors' response towards their queries regarding treatment. Further, it has been found that as the education level increases, the percentage of dissatisfied patients with doctors' response towards their queries also increases. As regards the cost involved in treatment, the study has shown that half of the patients have got information relating to expenses involved. However, they expressed that the information was provided only when they asked for it. It has also been found that the doctors do not explain to the patients about the surgical operation to be done and the risks involved before obtaining their consent, however, the patients wanted to get the adequate information about these aspects. The concept of 'informed consent' is found to be almost non-existent. Furthermore, there was dissatisfaction among the patients with the doctors' response towards their queries about the illness and the treatment. Thus, the doctors are lacking in providing the information to the patients about the illness, line of treatment and the cost involved, which is the root cause of patients' dissatisfaction.

Therefore, it is suggested that communication should be improved by considering patients as 'partners' in the process of treatment as has been advocated by the British Medical Association. The patients should be informed about the diagnosis, relevant investigations, necessary drug prescribed and the cost of treatment in a language understandable to them.

It is also suggested that the medical students at the undergraduate levels should be taught the communication skills and its importance. Effective patient-doctor communication can dispel uncertainty and fear and enhance healing and patient satisfaction. Since the main thrust of health care marketers is on patient satisfaction, it can be achieved by adopting 'patient-centered' approach by encouraging patients to ask questions, to seek a second opinion, and to share responsibility for medical decisions.

6.2.4 Accountability of the Doctors: As regards accountability of the doctors, the study has shown that more than half of the patients felt that the doctors did not feel accountable for their professional conduct. They were of the view that doctors should be accountable to general public, and this should be enforced through laws like the CPA.

However, a large majority of the doctors and the experts felt that the doctors were accountable for their professional conduct. While the doctors expressed that they were accountable to the Medical Council of India and the Indian Medical Association, majority of the experts felt strongly that the doctors must also be accountable to the Consumer Courts and to the Civil Courts.

6.2.5 Factors affecting Patients' Choice of a Hospital: The study has revealed that the patients choose a particular hospital mainly for the faith in and popularity of, the doctor. Convenient location, faith in and popularity of, the health institution and reasonable charges were also found to be the other factors for choosing a hospital. The study has further revealed that there are different reasons for choosing government and private health institutions. The major reasons for choosing a government hospital included referral by doctor and services provided free of cost. Faith in and popularity of the doctor and convenience of location were also found to be the major reasons for choosing a private health institution.

6.2.6 Patients' Expectations from Medical Profession: The major expectations of the patients from the medical profession were : immediate attention, proper diagnosis and sympathetic behaviour of the doctor. The doctors, too, appreciated the patients' expectations.

6.2.7 Perception about the Performance of Duties by Doctors: The study has shown that a whopping majority of the patients feel that some doctors are not doing justice to the patients while performing their duties. The opinion of the patients was substantiated by a large majority of the doctors and an overwhelming majority of the experts.

The top two reasons according to patients, doctors and experts included the commercialisation of the medical profession and the doctors' not feeling the necessity to provide information about the line of treatment to the patients.

However, the opinion of the patients and doctors of the government hospitals has reflected that the doctors in the government hospitals are overburdened with work and there are lack of proper facilities in the hospitals.

6.2.8 Actions Desired to be taken by Dissatisfied Patients: The study revealed that majority of the patients' who expressed dissatisfaction wanted to get compensation for damages suffered by them. A large majority of them complained to the hospital authorities. All of them were found to be dissatisfied with the remedial measures adopted by the hospital authorities. The study has further revealed that the dissatisfied patients favoured legal remedy under the Consumer Protection Act, 1986, as they considered it to be speedy, economical and involving minimum formalities in comparison to the Civil Courts. None of the patients expressed their opinion in favour of the Medical Council of India.

6.2.9 Patients' Awareness of CPA: The study has shown that even after a decade of its coming into force, the awareness of patients regarding the CPA is far from satisfactory. The remarks of Balachandran [1] that "consumer activist who happens to glance through the consumer grievances published in the media every week, will be shockingly disturbed to realise that even some of the educated, enlightened and otherwise well-informed consumers are neither aware of their rights as consumer nor of the existence of the Consumer Disputes Redressal Forums in the country", is supported by our findings. A large majority of the patients (79.6 percent) were found to be unaware of the CPA. Also, a large majority of graduates (82.4 percent) and even quite a large number of post-graduates and professionally qualified

(42.6 percent) were unaware of the CPA.

As the study revealed that a large majority of patients are grossly ignorant about the existence of various consumer grievance redressal agencies under the CPA, therefore, adequate consumer awareness should be created through consumer education. It is suggested that the Central and the State Consumer Protection Councils should take urgent steps towards creating awareness about the provisions of the CPA. The Central Government should make use of their Information and Broadcasting Department for this purpose. Voluntary consumer organisations should also come forward to supplement the government efforts in various ways, such as putting banners, placing of sign boards, distribution of brochures or through programmes in powerful media like television, and pamphlets giving necessary information about the various consumer forums whereby a consumer can file his complaints against deficiency in medical services.

For this purpose, voluntary consumer organisations need strengthening; and it is, therefore, necessary that the government provide adequate resources to registered voluntary consumer associations. In many countries where the consumer movement is at an advanced stage, the government provide financial and other support to consumer associations. The government of India should, therefore, evolve a sound policy of extending adequate financial aid to consumer associations. The Ministry of Civil Supplies, Consumer Affairs and Public Distribution of the Government of India, could be entrusted with the task of evolving guidelines for providing financial aid to registered voluntary consumer associations for effectively working for consumer protection.

In addition, the 'no fault' compensation programme, as has been adopted by the USA, Europe and New Zealand should be adopted in India also to provide a quick, cost-effective and fair means of compensating the victims of medical accidents. In this system, the victim does not have to prove in a court of law but has to pursue the appropriate board that the damage has resulted from someone else's negligence and has occurred in circumstances which qualify within the conditions laid down in the 'no fault' scheme. It could be beneficial to those whose injuries are serious, but do not wish to pursue compensation because they are unwilling to accept financial risks involved in the process. The necessary condition for a claim to qualify under the 'no fault' scheme is whether the injury could have been prevented by any alternative diagnostic or medical procedure or by performing the procedure differently. In this compensation is paid by the insurance company from a fund equally contributed by the doctor, health institution, patient and the government.

6.3 Doctors' and Experts' Viewpoints: CPA as a Means of Grievance Redressal Against Deficiencies in Medical Services

6.3.1 Awareness of Regulatory Measures for Medical Services: The study has revealed that a large majority of the doctors and all the experts were aware of the avenues available for action against deficiency of medical services including the Medical Council of India, the Indian Medical Association, the Civil Courts and the CPA, 1986. More than half of the doctors considered the Medical Council of India (MCI) to be the most appropriate avenue for taking action in the case of deficiency in medical services. They felt that medical technicalities of the case can be understood by medical experts only. However, a large majority of the experts favoured the CPA since they considered it to be speedy, economical and involving less formalities in comparison to the Civil Courts. The experts further expressed that since the Medical Council of India was mainly dominated by doctors, they were not sure that the patients could get proper justice.

Furthermore, the study has shown that a large majority of the doctors and a large majority of the experts found the legal measures including the Law of Torts, the Indian Penal Code and the Medical Council of India (MCI), not sufficient to provide redressal to patients' grievances as they are time consuming expensive and involved more procedural formalities and the MCI did not have provision to grant compensation to aggrieved patients.

While the amendment in the Indian Medical Council Act to provide compensation or amendment in the CPA to include medical expert was desired by the doctors, the experts favoured the CPA in its present form as a means of redressal of grievances against deficiency in medical services.

6.3.2 Desirability of Inclusion of Free Medical Services under the CPA: The opinion of a good number of doctors (both from government and private hospitals and private practitioners) and a whopping majority of the experts which include lawyers, judges, journalists, consumer activists and professors of law, indicates that medical services provided free of cost should also be covered under the CPA so that poor patients get redressal against medical negligence.

The study has shown that a whopping majority of the experts and a good number of doctors desired the inclusion of free medical services under the CPA. They expressed that people were paying taxes which was an indirect payment and further, poor people should also be allowed to sue against medical negligence and get compensation for the damage suffered by them.

The definition of the term 'service' under the CPA expressly excludes 'rendering of any service free of charge'. However it has been revealed that in many cases, the services provided by the Central and the State government hospitals to the patients free of charge were deficient, thereby resulting in loss or damage to consumer of such services. The present study has also shown that majority of the doctors and experts including lawyers, judges, journalists, consumer activists and professors of law favoured the inclusion of free medical services under the Act. It is, therefore, suggested that the concept of 'service' should be widened, and free medical services provided by the government hospitals or elsewhere be brought within the regulatory provisions of the Consumer Protection Act, by suitably amending the definition of 'service' given in the Act.

6.3.3 Redressal Mechanism under the CPA: The study has revealed that both the doctors and the experts in large majority felt that in comparison to the Civil Courts, the redressal under the CPA is speedy, inexpensive and involves minimum formalities.

6.3.4 Quality of Medical Service Provided and the CPA: The study has revealed that the application of the CPA to medical services would lead to improvement in the quality of medical services provided as the doctors would become careful towards their duties. Both the doctors and the experts in large majority expressed the same opinion on this aspect.

6.3.5 Perception About the Basis of Patient-doctor Relationship: The patient-doctor relationship was found to be based on mutual trust and faith. However, some experts also viewed it as a relationship where patient is a weaker party as doctors are experts in the field and the patients have to depend on them. Furthermore, the study has shown that the application of the CPA to medical services would not affect the relationship, in the long-run, though it may affect it in the short-run, as doctors may become apprehensive and resort to using defensive medical practices including asking for more pathological and other investigations, and buying medical indemnity insurance policies, leading to a substantial increase in the cost of treatment. The experts felt that the short-run effects would get neutralised in the long-run, thus relationship would not be affected. However, doctors did not agree with this view.

If the patient-doctor relationship is to be based on partnership and collaborated efforts as advocated by the British Medical Association, many of the disputes can be resolved at the preliminary level. It is, therefore, suggested that health care providers should adopt the 'partnership' concept, taking into consideration the needs and expectations of patients and their perception of medical services.

6.3.6 Necessity of Continuing Medical Education: The study has revealed the necessity of continuing medical education by all the doctors to update their knowledge in the medical field. Majority of the doctors expressed that in order to update their knowledge, they should subscribe medical journals, attend professional conferences and seminars and participate in training programmes. Further, they desired that a programme on developments in medical sciences, medical ethics, accountability and liability can be shown on the powerful medium like television. Therefore, it is suggested that the Indian Medical Association and the Medical Council of India should arrange seminars and workshops for the doctors. The main thrust should be on continuing medical education for updating the knowledge of the doctors with the recent developments which have taken place in the medical science, medical ethics, accountability and liability for medical negligence and the Consumer Protection Act, 1986.

6.3.7 Maintenance of Adequate Patients' Record: The study has revealed that a good number of doctors were not maintaining adequate records of their patients before the application of the CPA to medical services. However, in large majority, they expressed that doctors have started maintaining proper patients' records after the application of the CPA to the medical services. In the process doctors would become more careful regarding this aspect.

6.3.8 Implications of Application of CPA to Medical Services for Patient-doctor Relationship: The study has revealed that the application of CPA to medical services had certain implications including social, ethical, economic, and relating to medical education and profession, for the patient–doctor relationship.

The study has shown that with the application of the CPA to medical services, as held by the Supreme Court of India in 1995, the patients' awareness towards their right of quality medical care would increase. Doctors would be more careful in performing their duties. The doctors have expressed the possibility of doctors' suspecting patients as potential litigants and patients accusing doctors for every adverse outcome whereby patients conniving with lawyers to blackmail doctors. However, the experts have not shown agreement with doctors on these counts.

Regarding the ethical implications, the doctors felt that there might be hesitation on the part of the doctors in attending to serious and emergency patients and in using potentially risky procedures even in emergencies. Furthermore, the doctors would resort to defensive medicine including ordering of more investigations and tests just to play safe. However, the experts did not agree.

The study has further shown that both the doctors and experts are in agreement so far as the economic implications of the CPA to the patients are concerned. They expressed that the cost of increased investigation and the insurance premium would be ultimately passed on to the patients. However, the study has shown that it would also make doctors careful towards their training and education, in updating their knowledge and in maintaining adequate patients' records, thus improving the quality of medical service provided to patients. Thus, the study has shown a significant difference in the perception of the doctors and the experts in these regards.

6.4 CPA's Relevance for Patients' Grievance Redressal: The study has revealed that both the patients and the experts, in vary large majority found the Consumer Protection Act, 1986, to be helpful to patients in getting redressal of their grievances. However, the doctors were not found to be in agreement with the patients and the experts. More than half of the doctors felt that the applicability of the CPA to the medical services would lead to increased cost of treatment and practice of defensive medicine by the doctors, forcing patients to undergo unnecessary investigations. Thus, a note of optimism was expressed by the patients and experts that CPA would provide them succour by providing relief against deficiency in medical services.

Note

1. Balachandran, M.K. (1993), "Consumer Awareness in Consumer Protection", Upbhokta Jagran, March, p.7.

APPENDICES

Appendix 1
Medical Council of India
Code of Medical Ethics

The relevant parts of the 'Code of Medical Ethics', propounded by the Medical Council of India are reproduced below:

Declaration

At the time of registration, each applicant shall be given a copy of the following declaration by the Registrar concerned and shall read and agree to abide by the same :

1. I solemnly pledge myself to consecrate my life to the service of humanity;

2. Even under threat, I will not use my medical knowledge contrary to the laws of humanity;

3. I will maintain the utmost respect for human life from the time of conception;

4. I will not permit considerations of religion, nationality, race, politics or social standing to intervene between my duty and my patient;

5. I will practice my profession with conscience and dignity;

6. The health of my patient will be my first consideration;

7. I will respect the secrets which are confided in me;

8. I will give to my teachers the respect and gratitude which is their due;

9. I will maintain by all means in my power, the honour and noble traditions of the medical profession;

10. My colleagues will be my brothers;

I make these promises solemnly, freely and upon my honour.

Code

General Principles

1. *Character of the Physician*: The prime object of the medical profession is to render service to humanity; reward of financial gain is a subordinate consideration. Whosoever chooses this profession, assumes

the obligation to conduct himself in account with its ideals. A physician should be an upright man, instructed in the art of healing. He must keep himself pure in character and be diligent in caring for the sick. He should be modest, sober, patient, prompt to do his whole duty without anxiety; pious without going so far as superstition; conducting himself with propriety in his profession and in all the actions of his life.

2. *The Physician's Responsibility* : The principal objective of the medical profession is to render service to humanity with full respect for the dignity of man. Physicians should merit the confidence of patients entrusted to their care, rendering to each full measure of service and devotion. Physicians should try continuously to improve medical knowledge and skills and should make available to their patients and colleagues the benefits of their professional attainments. The physician should practice methods of healing founded on scientific basis and should not associate professionally with anyone who violates this principle. The honoured ideals of the medical profession imply that the responsibilities of the physician extend not only to individuals but also to society.

3. *Advertising* : Solicitation of patients directly or indirectly, by a physician, by groups of physicians or by institutions or organisations is unethical. A physician shall not make use of or aid or permit others to make use of him (or his name) as subject of any form or manner of advertising or publicity through lay channels, either alone or in conjunction with others which shall be of such a character as to invite attention to him or to his professional position, skill, qualification, achievements, attainments, specialities, appointments, associations, affiliations or honours and/or of such character as would ordinarily result in his self aggrandisement nor shall he give to any person whosoever, whether for compensation or otherwise, any approval, recommendation, endorsement, certificate, report or statement with respect of any drug, medicine, nostrum remedy, surgical or therapeutic article, apparatus or appliance or any commercial product or article with respect of any property, quality or use thereof or any test, demonstration or trial thereof, for use in connection with his name, signature, or photograph in any form or manner of advertising through lay channels nor shall be boast of cases, operations, cures or remedies or permit the publication of report thereof through lay channels. A medical practitioner is permitted a formal announcement in press regarding the

following:

(a) On starting practice
(b) On change of type of practice
(c) On changing address
(d) On temporary absence from duty
(e) On resumption of practice
(f) On succeeding to another practice

4. *Payment of Professional Services* : The ethical physician, engaged in the practice of medicine, limits the sources of his income received from professional activities to services rendered to the patient. Remuneration received for such services should be in the form and amount specifically announced to the patient at the time the service is rendered. It is unethical to enter into a contract of "no cure no payment".

5. *Patent and Copyrights* : A physician may patent surgical instruments, appliances and medicine or copyright publications, methods and procedure. The use of such patents or copyright or the receipt of remuneration from them which retards or inhibits research or restrict the benefits derivable therefrom are unethical.

6. *Running an open shop (Dispensing of drugs and appliances by Physicians)* : A Physician should not run an open shop for sale of medicine, for dispensing prescriptions prescribed by doctors other than himself or for sale of medical or surgical appliances. It is not unethical for a physician in prescribe or supply drugs, remedies or appliances as long as there is no exploitation of the patient.

7. *Rebates and Commission :* A Physician shall not give, solicit or receive any gift, gratuity, commission or bonus in consideration of or in return for the referring, recommending or procuring of any patient for medical, surgical or other treatment. A physician shall not directly or by any subterfuge participate in or by a party to the act of division, transference, assignment, subordination, rebating, splitting or refunding of any fee for medical, surgical or other treatment.

The provisions of this para shall apply with equal force to the referring, recommending or procuring by a physician or any person, specimen or material for diagnostic, or other study of work. Nothing in this section, however, shall prohibit payment of salaries by a qualified physician to other duly qualified person rendering medical care under his supervision.

8. *Secret Remedies* : The prescriptions or dispensing by a physician of secret medicine or other secret remedial agents of which he does not know the composition, or the manufacture or promotion of their use is unethical.

9. *Evasion of Legal Restrictions* : The physician will observe the laws of the country in regulating the practice of medicine and will not assist others to evade such laws. He should be co-operative in observance and enforcement of sanitary laws and regulations in the interest of public health. A physician should observe the provisions of the State Acts like Drugs Act, Pharmacy Act, Poisonous and Dangerous Drugs Act and such other Acts, Rules, Regulations made by the Central Government/State Governments or local Administrative Bodies for protection and promotion of public health.

Duties of Physicians to Their Patients

10. *Obligations to the Sick* : Though a physician is not bound to treat each and every one asking his services except in emergencies for the sake of humanity and the noble traditions of the profession, he should not only be ever ready to respond to the calls of the sick and the injured, but should be mindful of the high character of his mission and the responsibility he incurs in the discharge of his professional duties. In his ministrations, he should never forget that the health and the lives of those entrusted to his care depend on his skill and attention. A physician should endeavour to add to the comfort of the sick by making his visits at the hour indicated to the patients.

11. *Patience, Delicacy and Secrecy* : Patience and delicacy should characterise the physician. Confidence concerning individual or domestic life entrusted by patients to a physician and defects in the disposition or character of patients observed during medical attendance should never be revealed unless their revelation is required by the laws of the State. Sometimes, however, a physician must determine whether his duty to society requires him to employ knowledge, obtained through confidences to him as a physician, to protect a healthy person against a communicable disease to which he is about to be exposed. In such instance, the physician should act as he would desire another to act towards one of his own family in like circumstances.

12. *Prognosis* : The physician should neither exaggerate nor minimise the gravity of a patient's condition. He should assure himself

that the patient, his relatives or his responsible friends have such knowledge of the patient's condition as will serve the best interests of the patient and the family.

13. *The Patient Must Not be Neglected:* A physician is free to choose whom he will serve. He should, however, respond to any request for his assistance in an emergency or, whenever temperate public opinion expects the service. Once having undertaken a case, the physician should not neglect the patient, nor should he withdraw from the case without giving notice to the patient, his relatives or his responsible friends sufficiently long in advance of his withdrawal to allow them to secure another medical attendant. No provisionally or fully registered medical practitioner shall/will fully commit an act of negligence that may deprive his patient or patients from necessary medical care.

Appendix II
Hippocratic Oath

I swear by Apollo the physician, by Aesculapius, Hygiea and Panacea, and I take to witness all the gods, all the goddesses, to keep according to my ability and my judgement the following Oath:

"To consider dear to me as my parents him who taught me this art; to live in common with him and if necessary to share my goods with him; to look upon his children as my own brothers, and teach them this art if they so desire without fee or written promise; to impart to my sons and the sons of the master who taught me and the disciples who have enrolled themselves and have agreed to the rules of the profession, but to these alone, the precepts and the instruction. I will prescribe regimen for the good of my patients according to my ability and my judgement and never do harm to anyone. To please no one will I prescribe a deadly drug, nor give advice which may cause his death. Nor I will give a woman a pessary to procure abortion. But I will preserve the purity of my life and my art. I will not cut for stone, even for patients in whom the disease is manifest; I will leave this operation to be performed by practitioners (specialists in this art). In every house where I come I will enter only for the good of my patients, keeping myself far from all international ill-doing and all seduction, and especially from the pleasures of love with women or with men, be they free or slaves. All that may come to my knowledge in the exercise of my profession or outside of my profession or in daily commerce with men, which ought not to be spread abroad, I will keep secret and will never reveal. If I keep this oath faithfully, may I enjoy my life and practise my art, respected by all men and in all times; but if I swerve from it or violate it, may the reverse be my lot".

Appendix III
International Code of Medical Ethics

Duties of Doctors in General

A doctor must always maintain the highest standards of professional conduct.

A doctor must practise his profession uninfluenced by motives of profit.

The following practices are deemed unethical:

(a) Any self advertisement except such as is expressly authorised by the national code of medical ethics.

(b) Collaboration in any form of medical service in which the doctor does not have professional independence.

(c) Receiving any money in connection with services rendered to a patient other than a proper professional fee, even with the knowledge of the patient.

Any act or advice which could weaken physical or mental resistance of a human being may be used only in his interest.

A doctor is advised to use great caution in divulging discoveries or new techniques of treatment.

A doctor should certify or testify only to that which he has personally verified.

Duties of Doctors to the Sick

A doctor must always bear in mind the obligation of preserving human life.

A doctor owes to his patient complete loyalty and all the resources of his science. Whenever an examination or treatment is beyond his capacity he should summon another doctor who has the necessary ability.

A doctor shall preserve absolute secrecy on all he knows about his patients because of the confidence entrusted in him.

A doctor must give emergency care as a humanitarian duty unless he is assured that others are willing and able to give such care.

Duties of Doctors to Each Other

A doctor ought to behave to his colleagues as he would have them behave to him.

A doctor must observe the principles of The Declaration of Geneva approved by the World Medical Association.

Appendix IV

The Consumer Protection Act, 1986

(Act No. 68 of 1986) As amended by the Consumer Protection (Amendment) Act, 1993 (Act No. 50 of 1993)

An Act to provide for the better protection of the interests of consumers and for that purpose to make provisions for the establishment of consumer councils and other authorities for the settlement of consumers' disputes and for matters connected therewith.

Be it enacted by parliament in the Thirty-seventh Year of the Republic of India as follows:

1. **Short title, extent, commencement and application** - (1) This Act may be called the Consumer Protection Act, 1986.

2. It extends to the whole of India except the State of Jammu and Kashmir.

3. It shall come into force on such date as the Central Government may, by notification, appoint and different dates may be appointed for different States and for different provisions of this Act.

4. Save as otherwise expressly provided by the Central Government by notification. This Act shall apply to all goods and services.

2. **Definitions** - (1) In this Act, unless the context otherwise requires; -

(a) 'appropriate laboratory' means a laboratory or organisation -

(i) recognised by the Central Government;

(ii) recognised by a State Government, subject to such guidelines as may be prescribed by the Central Government in this behalf; or

(iii)any such laboratory or organisation established by or under any law for the time being in force, which is maintained, financed or aided by the Central Government or a State Government for carrying out analysis or test of any goods with a view to determining whether such goods suffer from any defect;

(aa) 'branch office' means -

(i) any establishment described as a branch by the opposite party; or

(ii) any establishment carrying on either the same or substantially the same activity as that carried on by the head office of the establishment; .

(b) 'complainant' means -

(i) a consumer; or

(ii) any voluntary consumer association registered under the Companies Act, 1956 (1 of 1956), or under any other law for the time being in force; or

(iii) the Central Government or any State Government;

(iv) one or more consumers, where there are numerous consumers having the same interest;

who or which makes a complaint;

(c) 'complaint' means any allegation in writing made by a complainant that -

(i) an unfair trade practice or a restrictive trade practice has been adopted by any trader;

(ii) the goods bought by him or agreed to be bought by him suffer from one or more defects;

(iii) the services hired or availed of or agreed to be hired or availed of by him suffer from deficiency in any respect;

(iv) a trader has charged for the goods mentioned in the complaint a price in excess of the price fixed by or under any Labour Organisation for the time being in force or displayed on the goods or any package containing such goods;

(v) goods which will be hazardous to life and safety when used are being offered for sale to the public in contravention of the provisions of any law for the time being in force requiring traders to display information in regard to the contents, manner and effect of use of such goods; with a view to obtaining any relief provided by or under this Act;

(d) 'consumer' means any person who -

(i) buys any goods for a consideration which has been paid or promised or partly paid and partly promised, or under any system of deferred payment and includes any user of such goods other than the person who buys such goods for consideration paid or promised or partly paid or partly promised, or under any system of deferred payment when such use is made with the approval of such person, but does not include a person who obtains such goods for re-sale or for any commercial purpose; or

(ii) hires or avails of any services for a consideration which has been paid or promised or partly paid and partly promised, or under any system of deferred payment and includes any beneficiary of such services other than the persons who hires or avails of the services for consideration paid or promised, or partly paid and partly promised, or under any system of deferred payment, when such services are availed of with the approval of the first mentioned person;

[Explanation - For the purposes of sub-clause (i), 'commercial purpose' does not include use by a consumer of goods bought and used by him exclusively for the purpose of earning his livelihood by means of self-employment].

(e) 'consumer dispute' means a dispute where the person against whom a complaint has been made, denies or disputes the allegations contained in the complaint;

(f) 'defect' means any fault, imperfection or shortcoming in the quality, quantity, potency, purity or standard which is required to be maintained by or under any law for the time being in force or [under any contract, express or implied, or] as is claimed by the traders in any manner whatsoever in relation to any goods;

(g) 'deficiency' means any fault, imperfection, shortcoming or inadequacy in the quality, nature and manner of performance which is required to be maintained by or under any law for the time being in force or has been undertaken to be performed by a person in pursuance of a contract or otherwise in relation to any service;

(h) 'District Forum' means a Consumer Disputes Redressal Forum established under clause (a) of Section 9.

(i) 'goods' means goods as defined in the Sale of Goods Act, 1930 (3 of 1930);

(j) 'manufacturer' means a person who -

(i) makes or manufactures any goods or parts thereof; of

(ii) does not make or manufacture any goods but assembles parts thereof made or manufactured by others and claims the end-product to be goods manufactured by himself; or

(iii) puts or causes to be put his own mark on any goods made or manufactured by any other manufacturers and claims such goods to be goods made or manufactured by himself.

[Explanation - Where a manufacture despatches any goods or part thereof to any branch office maintained by him, such branch office shall not be deemed to be the manufacturer even though the parts so despatched to it are assembled at such branch office and are sold or distributed from such branch office].

(jj) 'member' includes the President and a member of the National Commission or a State Commission or a District Forum as the case may be;

(k) "National Commission' means the National Consumer Disputes Redressal Commission established under clause (c) of Section 9;

(l) 'notification' means a notification published in the Official Gazette;

(m) 'person' includes -

(i) a firm whether registered or not;

(ii) a Hindu undivided family;

(iii) a co-operative society;

(iv) every other association of persons whether registered under the Societies Registration Act, 1860 (21 of 1860) or not.

(n) 'prescribed' means prescribed by rules made by the State Government or as the case may be, by the Central Government under this Act;

(nn) 'restrictive trade practice' means any trade practice which requires a consumer to buy, hire or avail of any goods, or, as the case may be, services as a condition precedent for buying, hiring or availing of other goods or services;

(o) 'service' means service of any description which is made available to potential users and includes the provision of facilities in connection with banking, financing, insurance, transport, processing, supply of electrical or other energy, board or lodging or both, [housing construction] entertainment, amusement or the purveying of news or other information, but does not include the rendering of any service free of charge or under a contract of personal service;

(p) 'State Commission' means a Consumer Dispute Redressal Commission established in a State under clause (b) of Section 9;

(q) 'trader' in relation to any goods means a person who sells or distributes any goods for sale and includes the manufacturer thereof, and where such goods are sold or distributed in package form, includes the packer thereof;

(r) 'unfair trade practice' means a trade practice which, for the purpose of promoting the sale, use or supply of any goods or for the provision of any service, adopts any unfair methods or unfair or deceptive practice including any of the following practices, namely -

1. the practice of making any statement, whether orally or in writing or by visible representation which -

(i) falsely represents that the goods are of a particular standard, quality, quantity, grade, composition, style or model;

(ii) falsely represents that the services are of a particular standard, quality or grade;

(iii) falsely represents any re-built, second-hand, renovated, reconditioned or old goods as new goods;

(iv) represents that the goods or services have sponsorship, approval, performance, characteristics, accessories, uses or benefits which such goods or services do not have;

(v) represents that the seller or the supplier has a sponsorship or approval or affiliation which such seller or supplier does not have;

(vi) makes a false or misleading representation concerning the need for, or the usefulness of any goods or services;

(vii) gives to the public any warranty or guarantee of the performance, efficacy or length of life of a product or of any goods that is not based on an adequate or proper test thereof:

Provided that where a defence is raised to the effect that such warranty or guarantee is based on adequate or proper test, the burden of proof of such defence shall lie on the person raising such defence;

(viii) makes to the public a representation in a form that

purports to be -

(i) a warranty or guarantee of a product or of any goods or services; or

(ii) a promise to replace, maintain or repair an article or any part thereof or to repeat or continue a service until it has achieved a specified result; if such purported warranty or guarantee or promise is materially misleading or if there is no reasonable prospect that such warranty, guarantee or promise will be carried out;

(ix) materially misleads the public concerning the price at which a product or like products or goods or services, have been or are, ordinarily sold or provided, and, for this purpose, a representation as to price shall be deemed to refer to the price at which the product or goods or services has or have been sold by sellers or provided by suppliers generally in the relevant market unless it is clearly specified to be the price at which the product has been sold or services have been provided by the person by whom or on whose behalf the representation is made;

(x) gives false or misleading facts disparaging the goods, services or trade of another person.

Explanation - For the purposes of clause (1), a statement that is -

(a) expressed on an article offered or displayed for sale, or on its wrapper or container; or

(b) expressed on anything attached to, inserted in, or accompanying an article offered or displayed for sale, or on anything on which the article is mounted for display or sale; or

(c) contained in or on anything that is sold, sent, delivered, transmitted or in any other manner whatsoever made available to a member of the public; shall be deemed to be a statement made to the public by, and only by, the person who had caused the statement to be so expressed, made or contained;

2. permits the publication of any advertisement whether in any newspaper or otherwise, for the sale or supply at a bargain price, of goods or services that are not intended to be offered for sale or supply at the bargain price, or for a period that is, and in quantities that are, reasonable, having regard to the nature of the market in which the business is carried on, the nature and size of business, and the nature of the advertisement.

Explanation - For the purposes of clause (2), 'bargaining price' means -

(a) a price that is stated in any advertisement to be a bargain price, by reference to an ordinary price or otherwise; or

(b) a price that a person who reads, hears or sees the advertisement, would reasonably understand to be a bargain price having regard to the prices at which the product advertised or like products are ordinarily sold;

3. permits -

(a) the offering of gifts, prizes or other items with the intention of not providing them as offered or creating impression that something is being given or offered free of charge when it is fully or partly covered by the amount charged in the transaction as a whole;

(b) the conduct of any contest, lottery, game of chance or skill, for the purpose of promoting, directly or indirectly, the sale, use or supply of any product or any business interest;

4. permits the sale or supply of goods intended to be used, or are of a kind likely to be used, by consumers, knowing or having reason to believe that the goods do not comply with the standards prescribed by competent authority relating to performance, composition, contents, design, constructions, finishing or packaging as are necessary to prevent or reduce the risk of injury, to the person using the goods;

5. permits the hoarding or destruction of goods, or refuses to sell the goods or to make them available for sale or to provide any service, if such hoarding or destruction or refusal raises or tends to raise or is intended to raise, the cost of those or other similar goods or services.

(2) Any reference in this Act to any other Act or provision thereof which is not in force in any area to which this Act applies shall be construed to have a reference to the corresponding Act or provision thereof in force in such area.

3. Act not in derogation of any other law - The provisions of this Act shall be in addition to and not in derogation of the provisions of any other law for the time being in force.

BIBLIOGRAPHY

A. Books

Aaker, David A. and George, S. Day (1971), *Consumerism : Search for the Consumer Interest* (New York : Free Press).

Advani, Rani (1990), *Consumer Protection Act and its Implications* (Ahmedabad: Consumer Education and Research Centre).

Advani, Rani (1991), *Patients : Know Yours Rights* (Ahmedabad : CERC).

Agarwal, V.K. (1997), *Consumer Protection in India* (New Delhi : Deep and Deep Publications).

Aggarwal, Anil and A.P. Chaudhari (1998), Medical Profession and the Consumer Protection Act (New Delhi : Aapee Publications Pvt. Ltd.).

Ahmad S.A (1994), The Fiduciary Concept : A Basis for an Ethics of Patient Care, *Souvenir,* (Medimeet, 1994, 23rd Assam State Medical Conference of Indian Medical Association, February 10-20, 1994, Nalbari, Assam).

American College of Physicians (1993), *Ethics Manual*, 3rd ed. (U.S.A. : ACP Ethics Committee, American College of Physicians).

American Medical Association (1992), *Code of Medical Ethics : Current Opinions* (Chicago : Council on Ethical and Judicial Affairs).

Anitia, N.H. and Kavita Bhatia (1993), *People's Health in People's Hand* (Bombay : The Foundation for Research in Community Health).

Asch, Peter (1988), *Consumer Safety Regulation* (New York : Oxford University Press).

Bailey, Kenneth, D. (1987), *Methods of Social Research*, 3rd ed. (New York : The Free Press).

Bakshi, P.M. (1993), *Law and Medicine* (Lucknow : Institute of Judicial Training and Research).

Basu, Durga Das (1996), *Constitution of India,* 12th ed. (New Delhi : Prentice Hall of India).

Borrie, Gorden J. and Aurbrey L. Diamond (1981), *Consumer, Society and Law*, 4th ed. (Harmondworth : Penguin).

Boyd, Harper W., Ralph Westfall and Stanley F. Stach (1977), *Marketing Research : Text and Cases* (Hornwood Illinois : Richard D. Irwin).

British Medical Association (1992), *Rights and Responsibilities of Doctors* (London : BMJ Publishing Group).

British Medical Association (1993), *Medical Ethics Today* (London : BMJ Publishing Group).

Charlesworth (1977), *Negligence,* 6th ed. (London : Sweet and Moxwell).

Chaudhari, R.S. (1993), *Doctor and the Consumer Protection Act* (Nasik : Maharashtra Law Agency).

Commonwealth Medical Association (1994), *Medical Ethics and Human Rights : Guiding Principles* (London : British Medical Association).

Consumers International (1996), *Compaigning for Patients Rights : A Consumer Action Kit* (London : Global Policy and Compaigns Unit).

Duggal, R. and Suchetha Amin (1988), *Cost of Health Care* (Pune : Foundation for Research in Community Health).

Feldman, Lawrence P. (1976), *Consumer Protection : Problems and Prospects* (St. Paul : West Publishing Co.).

Fisher, Fleur (1993), *Medical Ethics Today : Its Practice and Philosophy* (London : BMJ Publishing Group, BMA's Ethics, Science and Information Division).

Foundation for Research in Community Health (1997), *Health Care in India : A Profile* (Pune : FRCH).

Garg, O.P. (1991), *The Consumer Protection Act, 1986* (Delhi : Vinod Publishing House).

Goldring, J.L. and L.W. Maher (1979), *Consumer Protection Law in Australia* (Sydney : Butterworths).

Gorden, Raymond L. (1977), *Undimensional Scaling of Social Variables : Concepts and Procedures* (New York : The Free Press).

Green, Paul E. and Tull, Donald, S. (1986), *Research for Marketing Decisions* (New Delhi : Prentice Hall of India).

Grover, N.K. (1992), Consumer Protection Act : I.M.A. View Point, *Souvenir* (National Seminar on Problems of Medical Profession, organised by IMA, Moradabad).

Gulshan, S.S. (1994), *Consumer Protection and Satisfaction : Legal and Managerial Dimensions* (New Delhi : Wiley Eastern Limited).

IMA College of General Practitioners (1985), *Proceeding of National Workshop on Health Services Research* (New Delhi : IMA College of General Practitioners)

Indian Medical Association (1990), *Medical Ethics : An Update*, Proceedings of the National Seminar on Medical Ethics held at New Delhi on August 18-19, 1990 (New Delhi : An IMA Publication).

Indian Medical Association (1994), *Consumer Protection Act vis-à-vis Medical Profession : Stand of Indian Medical Association*, IMA's Policy Document, (New Delhi : IMA House).

Jesani, Amar and Shilpi Ganguli (1993), *Some Issues in Community Participation in Health Care Services* (Pune : FRCH).

Kalton, Graham (1983), *Introduction to Survey Sampling* (Beverly Hills, California : Sage Publication).

Kaushal A.K. (1995), *Medical Negligence and Legal Remedies with Special Reference to CPA Law* (New Delhi : Universal Book Traders).

Kotler, Philip (1997), *Marketing Management : Analysis, Planning, Implementation and Control*, 9th ed. (New Delhi : Prentice Hall of India).

Kramer, Charles (1968), *The Negligent Doctor* (New York : Crown Publishers).

Kress, George (1982), *Marketing Research* (Virginia : Reston Publishing Company).

Leehen, Henk, Sjef Gevers and Genevieve Pinet (1993), *The Rights of Patients in Europe : A Comparative Study* (Netherland : Kluwer Law and Taxation Publishers on behalf of WHO).

Leelakrishnan, P. (1990), *Consumer Protection and Legal Control* (Lucknow : Eastern Book Company).

Lele, R.D. (1992), *The Medical Profession and the Law* (Bombay : Sajjan Sons Publishers).

Mahalawar, K.P.S. (1991), *Medical Negligence and the Law* (New Delhi : Deep and Deep Publications).

Mukhopadhya, Alok (1992), *State of India's Health* (Delhi : Voluntary Health Association of India).

Nath, N.A. (1973), Unpublished M.D. thesis entitled "*A study of Central Government Health Science in Relation to Health Needs"* in Faculty of Medical Sciences, National Institute of Health and Family Welfare, University of Delhi, New Delhi.

Nathan, P.C. (1957), *Medical Negligence*, London.

Nijhawan, V.K. (1994), *Consumer Protection : Practice and Procedure* (Delhi : Vinod Publishing House).

Rohde, John, *et al.* (1993), *Reaching Health for All* (Oxford : Oxford University Press).

Rosenbloom, Larry J. (1981), *Consumer Complaint Guide* (New York : Macmillan Publishing Co.).

Sadananda, B. (1987), Unpublished M.D. thesis entitled "*A Study of Cost Analysis of Patients Care in a Large Hospital in Delhi*, in National Institute of Health Family Welfare, University of Delhi, New Delhi.

Sahni, Ashok (1995), *Legal Aspects of Health Care* (Bangalore : Indian Society of Health Administrators).

Saraf, D.N. (1990), *Law of Consumer Protection in India* (Bombay : N.M. Tripathi).

Satia, Harish Kumar (1986), unpublished M.D. thesis entitled "*A Study of the Factors Affecting the Out-patient Care as well as Effective Working of the Functional Dispensaries under ESI in Delhi*" in National Institute of Health and Family Welfare, University of Delhi, New Delhi.

Shah, K.K. and H.P. Mehta (1994), *Doctor and Law* (Ahmedabad : Silver Jubilee Publication of College of General Practitioner, edited by Dr. I.C. Shah, Gujrat State Branch, I.M.A.).

Shukla, V.N. (1994), *Constitution of India*, 9th ed. (Lucknow : Eastern Book Company)

Siegel, S. (1956), *Non-parametric Statistics for Behavioural Sciences* (New York : McGraw Hill).

Singh, Avtar (1994), *Law of Consumer Protection :* Principles and Practices (Lucknow : Eastern Book Company).

Singh, Gurbax (1991), *Law of Consumer Protection* (Jaipur : Bharat Law Publication).

Singh, Gurjeet (1996), *Law of Consumer Protection in India : Justice within Reach* (New Delhi : Deep and Deep Publications).

Singh, Jagdish (1994), *Medical Profession and Consumer Protection Act* (Jaipur : Bharat Law Publication).

Songuist, John A. and William C. Dunkelberg (1977), *Survey and Opinion Research : Procedures for Processing and Analysis* (New Jersey : Prentice Hall).

Sood, Kamlesh (1983), unpublished M.D. thesis entitled "*A Study of Quality of Health Services in Primary Health Centre Area*" in Community Health Administration, National Institute of Health and Family Welfare, University of Delhi, New Delhi.

Street, Harry (1972), *The Law of Torts*, 5th ed. (London : Butterworths).

Tandon, M.P. and Rajesh Tandon (1997), *The Indian Penal Code* (Faridabad : Allahabad Law Agency).

Timmappaya, A., *et al.* (1971), *Patient Satisfaction and Ward Social System*, National Institute of Health Family Welfare, Research Report No.3, pp.74.

Timmappaya, A., S. Chatopadhya, K.G. Agarwal and M. Advani (1973), *Hospital and its People*, National Institute of Health and Family Welfare, Report No.15, New Delhi.

Varma, P.S., M.S. Varma and Rajiv Sharan (1994), *Doctor and Consumer Protection Law* (Allahabad : Law Publications).

Voluntary Health Association of India (1992), *Medical Negligence : Issues Before the Public,* Health Action Series 3 (New Delhi : VHAI).

Voluntary Health Association of India (1995), *Health - Related Cases under Consumer Law* (New Delhi : VHAI).

Wani, V.R. and Girish Wani (1993), *Doctor in the Court* (Nashik : Maharashtra Law Agency).

Wheatley, Edward, W. (1983), *Marketing Professional Services* (Delhi : Prentice Hall of India).

Whincup, Michael H. (1980), *Consumer Legislation in the United Kingdom and the Republic of Ireland* (New York : Van Nostrand Reinhold Company).

World Health Organisation (1993), *Doctor–patient : Interaction and Communication* (Switzerland : Division & Mental Health, WHO).

World Health Organization (1998), *Global Health Law*, Proceedings, Selected Papers and Recommendations presented at the Inter-disciplinary International Conference on Global Health Law, New Delhi, 5-7 December, 1997, organised by Indian Law Institute, and WHO, Regional office for South East Asia, New Delhi (New Delhi : World Health Organisation).

Zeithaml, V.A., A. Parasuraman and L.L. Berry (1990), *Delivering Service Quality : Balancing Customer Perception and Expectations* (New York : The Free Press).

B. Articles

Aakar, David A. (1985), "Developing Effective Consumer Information Programmes", *Business Horizon,* Vol.25, No.1 (January-February), pp.32-39.

Advani, Poornima (1995), "Damocles Sword Over Doctors", *The Hindustan Times*, December 18, p.12.

Advani, Rani (1991), "The Consumer Protection Act, 1986 : Scope and Remedies", *Consumer Confrontation*, July-August, pp.52-54.

Aggarwal, K.K. (1996), "CPA : An Overview", *Indian Journal of Clinical Practice* (Speciality Issue on Medilaw), May, P.8.

Aggarwal, K.K. (1998), "At Crossroads", *The Hindustan Times*, Sunday Magazine, June 28, p.1, 4.

Agrawal, Manju, and Ajit K. Dalal (1994), "Patients in Indian Hospitals : Environmental Stresses and Affective Reactions", *The Indian Journal of Social Work*, January, pp.41-45.

Ahmed, Farooq (1994), "Amendments to Consumer Protection Act, 1986 : Some Subtle Aspects", *Consumer Protection Reporter*, Vol.1, No.4 (April), pp.900-904.

Anderson, Rolph E. and Marvin A. Jolson (1973), "Consumer Expectations and the Communication Gap", *Business Horizons*, Vol.16, No.2 (April) pp.11-16.

Asmslrong, David (1991), "What Do Patients Want?", *British Medical Journal*, Vol.303 (August 3), pp.26-27.

Bakshi, P.M. (1985), "Medicine, Law and Ethics : The Converging Frontiers", *World Congress on Law and Medicine, Souvenior*, New Delhi (February).

Bakshi, P.M. (1991), "Consumer Law and Voluntary Associations", *The Financial Express*, November 5, p.4.

Bal, Arun (1992), "Medical Councils : Failure to Enforce Code of Ethics", *Health for the Millions*, Vol.18, No.6 (December), pp.11-14.

Bal, Arun (1997), "Consumer Protection Act and Medical Profession", *Indian Pediatrics*, Vol.34 (April), pp.319-327.

Bal, Arun and Anil Pilgaonkar (1993), "Medical Records and Patients' Rights", *The Indian Journal of Social Work*, April, pp.189-192.

Banerjee, Ajay (1995), "Black Sheep among Docs will Stand Exposed", *The Tribune*, November16, p.3.

Barton, John M., *et al.* (1995), "The Compensation of Patients Injured in Clinical Trials", *Journal of Medical Ethics*, Vol.21, pp.166-169.

Baru, Rama (1994), "The Rise of Business in Medical Care", *Health for the Millions*, Vol.2, No.1 (February), pp.19-21.

Bas, A., Agbonifoh, and Pius E. Edorch (1980), "Consumer Awareness and Complaining Behaviour", *European Journal of Marketing*, Vol.20, pp.43-49.

Basu, Prabir (1995), "Damages and Compensation in COPRA", *Consumer Protection Reporter*, Vol.1, Part 3 (March), pp.477-78.

Behl, R.K. (1995), "Consumerism and Consumer Laws", *The Tribune*, March 15, p.7.

Berry, L.L., A. Parasuraman and V.A. Zeithaml (1988), "Service-Quality Puzzle" *Business Horizon*, September-October.

Bertia MMA Newsletter (1994), "Doctors in Private Hospitals", *Bertia MMA News Letter* (Malayasian Medical Association), Vol.25, No.8 (March) 8, p.5 (Editorial).

Bhasin, Ashok (1993), "Applicability of Consumer Protection Act to the Medical Profession", *Journal of the Indian Medical Association*, Vol.91 (July), p.193.

Bhatia, Sabina (1996), "Private Hospital devoid of Mercy" *The Hindustan Times*, July 8.

Bhatt, Kapil (1991), "Non-Judicial Machinery : Redressal of Complaints", *Consumer Confrontation*, July-August, p.49.

Bhatt, Kapil (1991), "The Consumer Protection Act, 1986 : Scope and Remedies", *Consumer Confrontation*, July-August, pp.50-51.

Bhattacharyya, Sourish and Sumit Ghosal (1995), "Physician Heal Thy Self", *The Times of India*, November 26, p.12.

Bopp, K.D. (1990), "How Patients Evaluate the Quality of Ambulatory Medical Encounters : A Marketing Perspective," *Journal of Health Care Marketing*, Vol.10, No.1, pp.6-16.

Boscarino, Joseph A. (1992), "The Public's Perception of Quality Hospital: Implication of Patients Survey's", *Hospital and Health Services Administration*, Spring, pp.13-35.

Boscarino, Joseph A. (1988) "The Public's Rating of Hospitals", *Hospital and Health Services Administration*, Vol.33 No.2 (Summer), pp.18-19.

Bose, N.S.C. (1992), "Medical Profession Not included under COPRA", *Health for the Millions*, Vol.18, No.6 (December), pp.15-17.

Brahams, D. (1987), "Medicine and Law : Doctors' Duty to Answer Patients' Inquiries", *The Lancet*, p.932.

Brailer, David J. and Lawrence Van Horn (1993), "Health and Welfare of US Business", *Harvard Business Review*, March-April, pp.125-132.

Brett, A.S. and L.B. Mc Cullough (1986), "When Patients Request Specific Intervention : Defining the Limits of Physician's Obligation", *New England Journal of Medicine*, Vol.315, No.21, pp.1347-1351.

Byrne, D.J., *et al.* (1988), "How Informed is Signed Consent", *British Medical Journal,* Vol.296 (March 19), pp.839-840.

Caplan, A.L. (1986), "Informed Consent", *The Lancet*, p.1160.

Carmel, Sara (1990), "Patient Complaint Strategies in a General Hospital", *Hospital and Health Services Administration*, Vol.35, No.2, pp.277-287.

Chengappa, Raj et al. (1993), "Medical Practices : Doctors in the Dock", *India Today*, June 15-30, pp.39-44.

Choudhuri, P.K. (1993), "Medical Profession and Consumer Protection Act", *Journal of the Indian Medical Association (JIMA)*, Vol.91, No.7 (July), pp.168-169.

Chowdhury, J. Roy (1994), "Doctor-Patient Relationship in a Multicultural Society", *The Journal of the Indian Medical Association (JIMA)*, Vol.92, No.12 (December), pp.413-414.

Chulani, H.C. (1999), "What is Medical Negligence?", *Physician's Digest*, Vol.8, No.1 (April-May), pp.43-48.

Churchill, G.A. and C. Suprenant (1982), "An Investigation into the Determinants of Customer Satisfaction", *Journal of Marketing Research*, Vol.19 (November), pp.491-504.

Clarke, Roberta, N. (1995), "Perception is Everything", *Journal of Health Care Marketing (A Quarterly Publication of American Marketing Association)*, Vol.15, No.3, pp.32-42.

Consumer Reports (1995), "How is Your Doctor Treating You?", Vol.60, No.2 (February), pp.81-86.

Contractor Munidhar C. (1990), "The Consumer Protection Act and its Implications", *Consumer Confrontation*, Issue No.78 (September-October), pp.29-32.

Contractor, Munidhar C. (1991). "Can Consumer Protection Act Cover Medical Services ?", *The Lawyers*, Vol.6, No.10 (October), pp.13-16.

Cunningham, William, H. Cunningham and C.M. Isabella (1976), "Consumer Protection : More Information or More Regulation?", *Journal of Marketing,* Vol.40 (April), pp.63-68.

David, Anthony (1996), "Stop! Wait a Minute!!", *Health Action*, Vol.9, No.2 (February), pp.4-5.

Dayal, Arvind (1994), "Legal Aspects of Health Care", *Indian Journal of Clinical Practice*, Vol.4, No.8 (January), pp.68-73.

Deva, M. Parameshvara (1994), "Ethics in Medicine", *Berita MMA Newsletter* (Malaysian Medical Association), Vol.25, No.8 (March), 8, p.1.

Dewan, Vijay Kumar (1991), "Consumers Should Wake Up and Assert their Legal Rights", *Consumer Protection Reporter (CPR)*, Vol.1, No.3 (March), pp.381-85.

Dewan, Vijay Kumar (1991), "Legal Protection for Consumers", *Consumer Protection Reporter* (CPR), Vol.2, No.9 (September), pp.349-53.

Duggal, Ravi, *et al.* (1995), "Health Expenditure across States : Part-I", *Economic and Political Weekly*, April, 15, pp.834-844.

Ellis, Chris (1995), "Doctor-Patient Relationship", *SA Family Practice* (Official Journal of the South African Academy of Family Practice and Primary Care), Vol.16, No.3 (March), pp.187-191.

Eradi, V.B. (1992), "Law is Here to Serve the Public", *Health for the Millions*, Vol.18, No.6, (December), pp.17-20.

Express News Service (1995), "Supreme Court Order Drives Doctors to Seek Insurance Cover", *Indian Express*, November, 16.

Fisk, T.A., C.J. Brown, K. Cannizzairo and B. Naftal (1990), "Creating Patients Satisfaction and Loyalty", *Journal of Health Care Marketing*, Vol.10, No.2, p.5-15.

Forvell, Class, and Robert A. Westbrook (1984), The Vicious Circle of Consumer Complaints" *Journal of Marketing*, Vol.48, pp.68-78.

Francis, C.M. (1996), "What We Need to Know about Consumer Protection Act, 1986 and Medical Negligence", *Health Action*, Vol.9, No.2 (February), pp.6-8.

Gae, Rustom S. (1993), "Consumer Protection and Medical Negligence", *Consumer Protection Judgements*, Vol.1, Part 1 (January), pp.1-9.

Gangadharan, K.R. (1993), "Winning Confidence and Avoiding Courts", *Health Action*, Vol.6, No.6 (June), pp.24-26.

Gelb, Betsy D., *et al.* (1988), "Service Marketing Lessons from the Professionals", *Business Horizons*, September–October.

George, Thomas (1996), "Informed Consent : A Pragmatic Approach", *Health For the Millions*, Vol.22, No.4 (July-August), p.10.

Gill, P.P.S. (1994), "Enactment of Law Not Enough", *The Tribune*, June 8, p.3.

Girimaji, Pushpa (1993), "Consumers Need Not Fear Section 26", *The Tribune*, October 8, p.10.

Girimaji, Pushpa (1994), "SC Verdict on CPA Awaited", *The Tribune*, February 25, p.10.

Girimanji, Pushpa (1994), "Bridging the Information Gap for Consumer : Consumer Protection", *Legal News and Views*, Vol.8, No.4 (April), pp.37-38.

Girimaji, Pushpa (1995), "Medical Negligence under the Consumer Protection Act", *The Times of India*, November 25, p.14.

Gleicher, N. (1984), "Caesarian Section Rates in United States : The Short Term Failure of the National Consensus Development Conference in 1980", *Journal of American Medical Association* (JAMA), Vol.252, pp.3273-3276.

Gokani A. (1995), "Doctors and Patients", *The Indian Express*, December. 25, p.8.

Gourisankar, V. (1993), "Bringing Doctors and Hospitals to Consumer Courts", *Health Action,* Vol.6 (June), pp.4-8.

Govindankutty, V. (1993), "The Consumer Protection Act and the Doctors", *Journal of the Indian Medical Association*, Vol.91 (July), pp.193-194.

Govindankutty, V. (1993), "Consumer Protection Act and The Medical Profession : A Critical Viewpoint", *Kerala Medical Journal (*KMJ*)*, Vol.34, No.2, pp.55-57.

Goyal, R.C. (1994), "Dilemma of Doctors and Patients", *Consumer Protection Judgements*, Vol.2, Part 3 (July), pp.13-21.

Grover, N.K. (1992), "Consumer Protection Act and Medical Profession", *IMA News*, April, pp.18-25.

Grover, N.K. (1993), "Accountability of Medical Professionals", *Journal of the Indian Medical Association (JIMA)*, October (Editorial).

Grover, N.K. (1998), "Doctor-Patient Relationship Today", *Karol Bagh Medical Association (KBMS) News Letter,* October.

Gulati, S.K. (1994), "Continuing Medical Education : The Need of the Hour", *Haryana Medical Journal*, March-April, pp.20-21.

Gupta, J.L. (1998), "Doctor in Consumer Act Web : Society's Restrained Response Needed", *The Tribune*, April 16.

Gupta, Rajesh (1995), "Redressal Agencies under the Consumer Protection Act, 1986 : Their Character, Scope of Power and Dominance over Domestic Tribunals : Some Issues", *Consumer Protection Judgements*, Vol.2, Part 1 (January), pp.1-10.

Gupta, Rajesh and Gunjan Gupta (1994), "Pervertive Professional and Perturbed Consumer : Dr. Subramanian's Case : A Critique", *Consumer Protection Judgements*, Vol.2, Part 4 (August), pp.33-44.

Gupta, Rajesh and Gunjan Gupta (1994), "Writ Jurisdiction of High Court under Consumer Protection Act : Dr. Subramanian's Case : An Eclipse?", *Consumer Protection Judgements*, Vol.3, Part 3 (November), pp.31-40.

Gupta, Shriniwas (1992), "Consumer Protection : Legislative Measures", *Yojna*, Vol.36, No.3 (February), pp.23-27.

Gupta, Shyam Sunder (1992), "Consumer Protection Act, 1986 : A Pragmatic Approach to Judicial Perestrioka", *Consumer Protection Reporter*, Vol.1, No.3 (March), pp.507-08.

Gupta, Shyam Sunder (1993), "Consumerism and Potential Users", *Consumer Protection Reporter*, Vol.1, No.3 (March), p.432.

Hariharan, R. (1990), "Consumerism Indian Style", *Indian Express*, January, p.4.

Harland, David (1991), "Implementing the Principles of the United Nations Guidelines for Consumer Protection", *Journal of the Indian Law Institute*, Vol.33, No.2 (April-June), pp.189-245.

Havard, John (1988), "*Ready, Steady,* GO : Making Doctors Complete", *British Medical Journal*, Vol.296 (April 2), pp.951-952.

Havard, John (1992), "No Fault Compensation for Medical Accidents", *Medical Science Law*, Vol.32, No.3, pp.187-198.

Heffring, Michael, P., *et al.* (1986), "High Tech, High Touch : Common Denomination in Patient Satisfaction", *Hospital and Health Services Administration*, Vol.33, No.2 (Summer), pp.189-198.

Hegde, B.M. (1996), "Medical Practice : Its Grey Areas", *Journal of Indian Medical Assocation (JIMA)*, Vol.94, No.12 (December), p.438 (Editorial).

Herzlinger, Regina E. (1989), "The Failed Revolution in Health Care : The Role of Management", *Harward Business Review*, March-April, pp.95-103.

Hill, C. Jeanne (1991), "Factors Influencing Physicians Choice", *Hospital and Health Services Administration*, Winter, pp.491-503.

Himachalam, D. (1990), "Consumerism in India", *Indian Journal of Marketing*, Vol.20, No.6 (February), pp.7-10.

Indian Express (1995), "Doctors Upset by SC Verdict", November 16.

Indian Medical Tribune (1994), "Medical Care Guidelines : Preaching Practice Norms to Doctors", *Indian Medical Tribune*, March 15, Section 3, p.10.

Inquanzo, Joe M. and Mark Harju (1985), "Consumer Satisfaction with Hospitalization", *Hospitals*, May 1, pp.81-84.

Iyer, Aditi, (1996), "Crisis of Credibility : The Tale of Medical Councils", *Health for the Millions*, Vol.22, No.4 (July-August), pp.17-20.

Iyer, V.R. Krishna (1992), "Consumer Protection and the Medical Profession", *The Hindu*, July 7, p.10..

Jain, Kalpana (1995), "Malpractice Cases will Speed Up", *The Hindustan Times*, November 28.

Jalgaonkar, Mangesh (1994), "Consumer Protection Act : An Introspection by a General Practitioner", *Journal of Forum for Medical Ethics*, Vol.2, No.2 (November-December), pp.12-13.

James, Ahraham, J. (1993), "Consumer Protection Not for Doctors Forum!!!," *Journal of the Indian Medical Association* (JIMA), Vol.91 (July), p.193.

Jena, K.N. (1995), "Role of Members of Redressal Agencies for Effective Implementation of Consumer Protection Act, 1986", *Consumer Protection Judgements*, Vol.1, Part 1 (January), pp.10-16.

Jesani, Amar (1993), "Medical Ethics and Patients' Rights", *The Indian Journal of Social Work*, April, pp.173-188.

Jesani, Amar and Vimla Nandkani (1993), "Patients' Rights : A Perspective", *The Indian Journal of Social Work* (Tata institute of Social Sciences), April, pp.167-171.

John, Wilson (1995), "Docs in the Dock", *The Hindustan Times*, November 22, p.1.

Joseph, John (1993), "Consumer Revolution", *The Hindustan Times*, May 15, p.9.

Joshi, Poornima (1999), "Lack of Clear Policy and Planning hits Health Care Sector", *The Hindustan Times,* Lifeline, March 9.

Joshi, Poornima and Rema Nagarajan (1999), "Trans-Yamuna Health Care Pathetic", *The Hindustan Times* (Lifeline), February 28, p.3.

Kalafat, John (1991). "A Systematic Health Care Quality Service Program", *Hospital and Health Services Administration*, Vol.36, No.4, pp.571-586.

Kenneth, E. Clow, Arthur Fisher and David O' Bryan (1995), "Patient Expectations of Dental Services, *Journal of Health Care Marketing* (A Quarterly Publication of American Marketing Association), Vol.15, No.3.

Khan, Sameera (1995), "Doctors must Take the Rap", *The Times of India*, December 10, p.5.

Kohli, P.K. (1994), "CPA : Let us Face it," *Haryana Medical Journal*, March-April, pp.24-28.

Kotler, Philip (1972), "What Consumerism Means for Marketers", *Harvard Business Review*, Vol.50, No.3(May-June), pp.48-57.

Kotler, Philip and Richard A. Connor (1977), "Marketing Professional Services", *Journal of Marketing*, January, pp.71-76.

Kovner, Anthony R. (1991), "The Case of the Unhealthy Hospital", *Harvard Business Review*, September-October, pp.12-26.

Krishna, Bal (1995), "SC Ruling on Doctors a Welcome Step", *The Hindustan Times*, November 30, p.9.

Kumar, Parveen (1992), "Patients can Sue Doctors under Consumer Protection Act, 1986", *Consumer Protection Reporter*, Vol.2, No.7 (July), pp.70-73.

Kuppuswamy, Alladi (1993), "Balancing between the Rights of the Doctor and the Rights of the Patient", *Health Action*, Vol.6, No.6 (June), pp.9-13.

Lamont, Linda (1994), "When Things Go Wrong", *ODA News Review (Overseas Doctors' Association)*, Vol.3, Issue No.12 (March-April), pp.11-17.

Lanning, Joyce A. (1990), "The Health Care Quality Quagmire : Some Signposts", *Hospital and Health Services Administration*, Vol.35, No.1, pp.39-42.

Lum, Milton (1998), "The Black Sheep of the Medical Profession", *Bertia MMA News Letter* (A Newsletter of Malaysician Medical Association), Vol.28, No.3 (March), p.3.

Lum, Milton (1998), "The Principles of Managed Care", *Bertia MMA News Letter* (A Newsletter of Malaysician Medical Association), Vol.28, No.3 (March), p.15.

Malhotra, Preeti (1996), "Hospital Gasping for Breath", *The Hindustan Times* (*The Metropolitan*), October, 9, p.1.

Mathew, N.M. (1996), "When Complaints are Frivolous", *Health Action*, Vol.9, No.2 (February), pp.23, 40.

Mathew, N.M. (1997), "Quality Health Care : A Mirage or Reality", *Health for the Millions*, March-April, pp.37-39.

McCoy, R.S. (1998), "Social Responsibility and the Physician", *Bertia MMA News Letter* (A News Letter of Malaysician Medical Association), Vol.28, No.3 (March), pp.1, 12-13.

Mehta, P. (1992), "Do Doctors have a License to Kill?", *Health for the Millions*, Vol.18, No.6 (December), pp.7-10.

Mehta, R.R.S. (1988), "Personal Banking Services : UK Examples", *Prajnan*, June, pp.235-239.

Meisel, Alan and Mark Kuczewki (1998), "Legal and Ethical Myths about Informed Consent", *Bertia MMA News Letter* (A Newsletter of Malaysician Medical Association), Vol.28, No.3 (March), pp.16-17.

Menon, N.R. Madhava (1993), "Strengthening Self-Regulation in the Medical Profession for the Health of All", *Health Administrator* (Official Publication of the Indian Society of Health Administrators), Vol.4, No.2 (December).

Mittal, N.K., Batra, R., *et al.* (1996), "CPA Presented as a Syndrome", *Journal of the Indian Medical Association*, Vol.94, No.11, p.425-425.

Mohamed, N.S. (1996), "Professionalising Service Marketing", *Indian Journal of Marketing*, Vol.25, No.56 (May–June), pp.17-20.

Mohan, Pradeep (1990), "Professional Negligence", *Haryana Medical Journal*, Vol.10, No.12, pp.277-281.

Mohan, Sadhna (1991), "Strong Medicine", *The Times of India*, February 16.

Munidhar, C. (1993), "Can the Consumer Protection Act, 1986 Encompass Medical Service?", *Journal of the Indian Medical Association*, Vol.91 (July), pp.194-195.

Murty, O.P. (1996), "Caution to Medical Practitioner", *Indian Journal of Clinical Practice*, Speciality issue on Medilaw, May, pp.31-33.

Nagarajan, S. (1994), "Doctor and the Law", *SIMA News*, Publication of the Indian Medical Association, Salem Branch, February, pp.4-16.

Narayan, Ravi (1987), "More Powers for MCI", *Economic and Political Weekly*, Vol.22, September 26, pp.16, 22-33.

Navrange, Jayant (1994), "CPA and Doctors", *Imates (Newsletter of Indian Medical Association, Pune Branch*), Vol.7, No.4 (January), pp.6-8.

Nelson, Carl, W. (1990), "Patients' Satisfaction Survey : An Opportunity for Total Quality Improvement", *Hospital and Health Services Administration*, Vol.35, No.3 (fall), pp.409-427.

Orme, Clifton, N. (1992), "Customer Information and the Quality Improvement Process : Developing a Customer Information System", *Hospital and Health Services Administration*, Vol.37, No.2, pp.197-212.

Padamanabhan, B.S. (1991), "Redress Machinery is Deficient : Interview with H.D. Shourie", *Frontline*, Vol.8, No.24 (December 6), pp.86-87.

Pandya, Sunil K. (1993), "The Rights of Patients", *The Indian Journal of Social Work*, April, pp.205-208.

Pandya, Sunil K. (1995), "Doctor-patient Relationship", *Medical Ethics*, Vol.3, No.2 (April-June), p23.

Parasuraman, A., *et al.* (1985), "A Conceptual Model of Service Quality and its Implication for Future Research", *Journal of Marketing*, Fall, pp.41-50.

Phatnani, Pritam P. (1995), "Medico-Legal Aspects of Doctor-Patient Relationship", *Express Pharma Pulse*, November, 30, pp.5-6.

Pilgaokar, Anil (1996), "Doctors and the Consumer Protection Act", *Medical Ethics*, Vol.4, No.1 (January–March), p.2.

Potdar, Ramesh D. (1997), "Consumer Protection Law and Pediatrician", *Indian Pediatrics*, Vol.34 (April), pp.283-286.

Quam, L., R. Dingwall and P. Fenn (1987), "Medical Malpractice in Perspective : The American Experience", *British Medical Journal*, June, pp.1529-1531.

Rahman, M. (1993), "Consumer Courts : Power to the People", *India Today*, January15, pp.100-101.

Rama, Rao, P.S. (1984), "Consumer Protection : Myths or Reality ?", *Indian Journal of Marketing*, Vol.14, No.7 (March).

Raveendran, Basu (1996), "Ethical Committee Speaks", *News Letter of I.M.A. Kerala State*, January, p.3.

Ray, D.B. (1974), "A Study of Opinions of Patients to Measure Level of Satisfaction", *National Institute of Health and Family Welfare Bulletin*, Vol.7, No.3, pp.171-185.

Ray, Inderjit (1996), "Doctor-Patient Relationship in the Hospital", *Editorials of JIMA on Medico-social Issues, January 1931 – September 1996, Journal of the Indian Medical Association*, p.92.

Reynolds, R.A., J.A. Rizzo and M.L. Gorgalez (1987), "The Cost of Medical Professional Liability", *Journal of American Medical Association* (JAMA), Vol.257, pp.2276-2781.

Rhee, Sang O. (1976), "Factors Determining the Quality of Physicians' Performance in Patient-Care" *Medical Care*, Vol.14, No.9 (September), pp.733-750.

Ross, H.R. (1985), "Customer Service in a Hospital Out-Patient Department", *Hospital and Health Services Administration*, November, pp.274-277.

Sachdeva, M. (1993), "Medical Ethics : Role of Medical Council of India", *New Delhi Medicos*, (An Official Journal of IMA, New Delhi Branch), Vol.9, No.12 (December), pp.20-24.

Sachdeva, M. (1993), "Medical Negligence", New *Delhi Medicos* (Official Journal of IMA, New Delhi Branch), Vol.9, No.12 (December), pp.19-20.

Sachdeva, T.R. and Tripta Bhasin (1983), "Hospital and Society and their Expectations", *Swasth Hind* (Central Health Education Bureau), September, pp.225-228.

Sahni, Ashok (1994), "Consent in Medical Care", *Health Administrator* (Official Publication of the Indian Society of Health Administrators, Bangalore), Vol.5, No.1 (July), pp.152-155.

Sahu, G.N. (1981), "Consumer Problems in India", *Indian Journal of Marketing*, Vol.2, No.9 (May), pp.26-29, 34.

Sander, A.A. (1957), "The History of Professional Liability Suits in the United States" *Journal of American Medical Association*, Vol.163, No.6, pp.459-466.

Sandrick, Karen (1986), "Quality : Will it Make or Break Your Hospital", *Hospitals*, July 5, pp.54-58.

Sangwan, Soni (1998), "Diagnostic Centres make Hay as Government Hospitals Give Way", *The Hindustan Times*, Lifeline, March 6.

Sangwau, Soni (1996), "Was it callous Negligence ? : Fatal Punch for Army Cadet", *The Hindustan Times*, April 20, p.3.

Saraf, D.N. (1992), "Genesis of COPRA" *Health for the Millions*, Vol.18, No.6 (December), pp.21-24.

Sastry, T. Suryanarayan (1992), "The Role of the Voluntary Organisations in Creating Consumer Awareness", *All India Reporter*, Vol.79, Part 942 (June), pp.89-90.

Save, Sudhakar and R.V. Govani (1999), "Informed Consent", *Gujarat Medical Journal*, Vol.56, No.1 (February) pp.48-54.

Sawarkar, J.G. (1996), "Consumer Awareness : A Survey Analysis", *Indian Journal of Marketing*, Vol.25, No.10 (October-November), pp.13-21.

Shaber Ali, G. (1992), "Negligence of Doctors : Whom Should the Victim Approach ?", All India Reporter, Vol.79, Part 946 (October), pp.148-52.

Sharma, Kalpana (1994), "The Rot in the Medical System", *Health Administrator* (Official Publication of the Indian Society of Health Administrators, Bangalore), Vol.5, No.1 (July), pp.156-159.

Sharma, R.D. (1995), "Pros and Cons of SC Judgement", *The Hindustan Times*, November 29, p.13.

Shourie, H.D. (1991), "Raw Deal for Consumers", *The Economic Times*, April, p.4.

Shourie, H.D. (1993), "Doctors and Patients : A Sacred Tie", *The Hindustan Times*, August, 19, pp.12-13.

Simanowitz, Arnold (1985), "Standards, Attitudes and Accountability in the Medical Profession", *The Lancet*, September 7, pp.546-547.

Singh, B.N.P. (1993), "Impact of Consumer Protection Act on Medical Practice", *Health Administrators*, Vol.4, No.2 (December), pp.56-61.

Singh, Puspa and Hem Chandra (1998), "Citizen Charter versus Medical Ethics and Health Legislation", *Journal of Indian Medical Association (JIMA), Calcutta* Branch, Vol.96, No.9 (September), pp.282, 287.

Singh, R. (1990), "Consumers' Attitude towards Consumerism : An Exploratory Study", *Consumer Confrontation,* Vol.10, No.1, pp.8-11.

Suryanarayana (1992), "The Role of The Voluntary Organisations in Creating Consumer Awareness", *All India Reporter*, Vol.79, Part 942 (June), pp.89-90.

Taylor, P.W. and Nelson E., *et al.* (1981), "Development and Use of a Method of Assessing Patients' Perception of Care" *Hospital and Health Services Administration*, Winter, pp.89-104.

Taylor, Steven, A. (1994), "Distinguishing Service Quality from Patient Satisfaction in Developing Healthcare Marketing Strategies". *Hospital and Health Services Administration*, Vol.39, No.2 (Summer), pp.221-236.

Taylor, Steven, A., and Joseph J. Cronin, (1994), "Modeling Patient Satisfaction and Service Quality" *Journal of Health Care Marketing,* Vol.14 (Spring), pp.34-44.

The Hindustan Times, Parliament News (1992), "Health Service under Consumer Protection Act Likely", April 11.

The Hindustan Times (1993), "Medical Profession : Consumer Act may Act as Deterrant", April 12, p.7.

The Times of India (1995), "Doctors can't Loot and Scoot Forever : Interview with Dr. N.H. Anitia", November 18, p.2.

Thiagarajan, K. (1981), "An Ombudsman for the Consumer", *The Financial Express*, July 6, p.5.

Thukral, Naveen (1995)," Doctors Sceptical as Patients Hails Verdict", *The Indian Express*, November 16, p.6.

Tiwari, O.P. (1991), "Appeals under the Consumer Protection Act 1986", *Consumer Protection Reporter*, Vol.1, No.2, pp.209-213.

Tiwari, O.P. (1991), "Complaints and Reliefs in the Consumer Forums of India", *Consumers Protection Reporter*, Vol.1, No.2, pp.209-13.

Turner, Paul D. and L.G. Pol (1995), "Beyond Patient Satisfaction", *Journal of Health Care Marketing (AMA)*, Vol.15, No.3, pp.45-53.

Unnikrishnan, P.V. and R.V. Baru (1992), "Consumer Protection Act", *Health for the Millions*, Vol.18, No.6 (December), pp.2-6.

Vardhan, R. Yashod (1994), "Medical Negligence and Consumer Fora : The Tussle Continues", *The Lawyers* (The Lawyers Collective Publication, Bombay), May, pp.26-27.

Vaz, Walter (1996), "COPRA : Primordial Prevention and Pre-emption", *Indian Journal of Clinical Practice (IJCP)*, Speciality Issue on Medilaw, May, pp.35-37.

Venugopal, S. (1994), "Accused' Overseas Doctors Need Special Protection Until Proven Guilty", *ODA News Review*, Vol.3, Issue No.12 (March-April), p.9.

Verma, D.P.S. (1984), "Consumer Protection : Problems and Prospects", *The Economic Times*, June, 16.

Verma, D.P.S. "The Consumer Protection Act : A New Challenge to the Marketing Manager", a paper presented at the faculty seminar on "Business Strategy in Regulated Environment", New Delhi, March, 1987.

Wexler, Robert (1973), "Court Ordered Consumer Arbitration", *The Arbitration Journal*, Vol.28, pp.175-184.

Woodside, A.G., L.L. Frey and R.T. Daly (1989), "Linking Service Quality, Customer Satisfaction, and Behavioural Intention," *Journal of Health Care Marketing,* Vol.9, No.4, pp.5-17.

Xirasagar, Sudha (1993), "Patients' Right of Access to Health Records ?", *Health Administrators*, Vol.4, No.2 (December), pp.46-47.

Yadwad, B.S. (1993), "Consumer Protection Act and the Medical Profession", *Health Administrators,* Vol.4, No.2 (December), pp.51-54.

Zachary (1975), "Consumer Protection", *Indian Journal of Marketing,* Vol.5, pp.25-26.

C. Reports

Government of India, *Gazette of India (Extra Ordinary),* Part II, Section 1, No.83, dated December 26, 1986.

Government of India, Ministry of Health and Family Welfare, *Health Information of India : 1991,* Director General of Health Services, G.K. Vishwakarma, New Delhi, 1992.

Government of India, *Gazette of India (Extra Ordinary),* Part II, Section 1, No.84, dated June 18, 1993.

Government of India, *Health Information of India*, Ministry of Heath and Family Welfare, New Delhi, 1993.

Government of India, Ministry of Civil Supplies, Consumer Affairs and Public Distribution, *Directory of Voluntary Consumer Organisations,* New Delhi, 1993.

Government of National Capital Territory of Delhi, Directorate of Health Services, *Medical Directory*, New Delhi, 1992.

United Nation's Development Programme (UNDP), *Human Development Report* 1995, Oxford University Press, Delhi, 1995.

World Bank, *World Development Report 1993 : Investing in Health*, Oxford University Press, New York, 1993.

Index

A
American Medical Association, 9
Approach of the consumer courts, 110

B
Babylonian laws of Hummarabi, 9
British Medical Association, 6

C
Care provided in operation, 239
Central Consumer Protection Council, 83
Code of Medical Ethics, 6
Commonwealth Medical Association, 6
Consumer Protection Act, 1986, 63
Consumer Protection Bill, 1986, 63
CPA's role in grievance redressal, 263

D
Defensive medicine, 50
Delhi State Commission, 271
Doctors' professional accountability, 249

E
Express consent, 22

F
Functioning of the consumer courts, 106

G
Government servants under CGHS, 81
Gross negligence in medical services, cases, 136

H
Hippocratic Oath, 9

I
Implied consent, 22
Indian Contract Act, 1972, 8
Indian Medical Association, 4
Indian Medical Council Act, 1956, 62
Indian Penal Code, 1860, 60
Information regarding treatment, 224
Informed consent, 22

L
Law of torts, 61

M

Maintenance of patients' records, 265
Medical audit, 29
Medical negligence, liabilities for, 19
Medical negligence, types of, 18
Medical Ombudsman, 31
Medical services, deficiency in, 24

N

National Commission, 90
Negligence not established, cases, 142
No fault compensation programme, 32

O

Opportunity given to produce evidence, cases, 141

P

Patient-centred approach, 28
Patients' dissatisfaction, reasons for, 276
Patients' satisfaction with OPD services, 274
Perceived injustice to patients by doctors, 247
Proxy consent, 24

Q

Quality control circles, 30
Quality of patients' care, 47

R

Reduction of compensation. cases, 134
Resjudicata, 72

S

Sample doctors, profile of, 243
Sample experts, profile of, 245
Sample patients, profile of, 211
Seeking expert opinion, cases, 139
Side-effects of prescribed drugs, 249
State Commission, 88

V

Vicarious liabilities, 20
Voluntary Health Association of India, 2

W

World Consumer Rights Day, 3
World Health Organisation, 1